Fast Facts

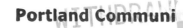

# Fast Facts:
# Asthma

Fourth edition

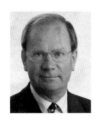

**Stephen T Holgate** MD DSc FRCP FMedSci
MRC Clinical Professor of Immunopharmacology
School of Medicine
Southampton General Hospital
Southampton, UK

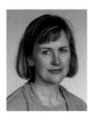

**Jo A Douglass** MB BS MD FRACP
Head, Department of Clinical Immunology and Allergy
Royal Melbourne Hospital
Honorary Clinical Professor, University of Melbourne
Parkville, Victoria, Australia

**Declaration of Independence**
This book is as balanced and as practical as we can make it.
Ideas for improvement are always welcome: feedback@fastfacts.com

HEALTH PRESS

Fast Facts: Asthma
First published 1999; second edition 2006; reprinted 2007; third edition 2010
Fourth edition March 2013

Text © 2013 Stephen T Holgate, Jo A Douglass
© 2013 in this edition Health Press Limited
Health Press Limited, Elizabeth House, Queen Street, Abingdon,
Oxford OX14 3LN, UK
Tel: +44 (0)1235 523233
Fax: +44 (0)1235 523238

Book orders can be placed by telephone or via the website.
For regional distributors or to order via the website, please go to:
fastfacts.com
For telephone orders, please call +44 (0)1752 202301 (UK, Europe and Asia–
Pacific), 1 800 247 6553 (USA, toll free) or +1 419 281 1802 (Americas).

Fast Facts is a trademark of Health Press Limited.

A CIP record for this title is available from the British Library.

ISBN 978-1-908541-13-0

Holgate ST (Stephen)
Fast Facts: Asthma/
Stephen T Holgate, Jo A Douglass

Medical illustrations by Dee McLean and Jane Fallows, London, UK.
Typesetting and page layout by Zed, Oxford, UK.
Printed by Latimer Trend & Company, Plymouth, UK.

Text printed on biodegradable and recyclable paper
manufactured using elemental chlorine free (ECF) wood pulp
from well-managed forests.

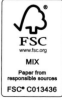

FSC
www.fsc.org
MIX
Paper from
responsible sources
FSC® C013436

# Glossary

**AMP:** adenosine 5'-monophosphate

**ASA:** acetylsalicylic acid (aspirin)

**Atopy:** a condition characterized by excessive production of immunoglobulin (Ig)E in response to allergens

**Basophil:** a type of white blood cell, distinguishable on staining

**B lymphocyte:** a type of white blood cell that produces antibodies

**COPD:** chronic obstructive pulmonary disease

**CysLTs:** cysteinyl leukotrienes, a powerful class of bronchoconstricting mediators

**Cytokine:** a peptide secreted by cells involved in inflammation and the immune response; cytokines can control the activity and growth of the cell that secreted them, or nearby cells

**Daily variability:** variability in daily peak expiratory flow (PEF), calculated as a percentage of the mean daily PEF value

**DPI:** dry-powder inhaler

**Eosinophil:** a type of white blood cell involved in allergic responses, distinguishable on staining

**FEV$_1$:** forced expiratory volume in 1 second, a measure of lung function

**FVC:** forced vital capacity, a measure of lung function

**GINA:** Global Initiative for Asthma, an international scientific initiative created to provide and encourage the use of scientific reports on asthma and asthma research

**IFNγ:** interferon-γ, a cytokine that has the capacity to inhibit the development of the allergic pathways, under normal conditions

**IgE:** immunoglobulin class E, a class of antibody secreted by B lymphocytes on exposure to allergen; binding of IgE to certain cells involved in the immune response results in the release of inflammatory mediators

**IL:** interleukin, a cytokine that controls a specific aspect of hemopoiesis or the immune response

**LABA:** long-acting β$_2$-agonist

**Leukocyte:** white blood cell

**Mast cell:** a large cell containing chemical mediators that are released in inflammatory and allergic responses

**MDI:** metered-dose inhaler

**NSAID:** non-steroidal anti-inflammatory drug

**$Pa$CO$_2$:** partial pressure of carbon dioxide in arterial blood

**$Pa$O$_2$:** partial pressure of oxygen in arterial blood

**PEF:** peak expiratory flow, a measure of lung function

**pMDI:** pressurized metered-dose inhaler

**SABA:** short-acting β$_2$-agonist

**SpO$_2$:** oxygen saturation measured by pulse oximeter

**T lymphocyte:** a type of white blood cell that is mainly responsible for cell-mediated immunity

**Th lymphocyte:** T helper lymphocyte; a type of T lymphocyte that is activated on exposure to allergen and releases cytokines

**Trigger:** a stimulus that increases asthma symptoms and/or airflow limitation

# Introduction

Asthma affects over 20 million people worldwide, with a large individual, social and economic burden of disease. In developed countries, severe and difficult asthma remains a stubborn problem in terms of healthcare costs, pressure on healthcare providers and individual quality of life. In low- and middle-income countries, especially those adopting aspects of Western lifestyles rapidly, asthma and associated allergy are increasing in prevalence, while high mortality rates point to inadequate diagnosis and lack of use of proven effective asthma treatments.

This fully updated fourth edition of *Fast Facts: Asthma* incorporates several new perspectives. Effective asthma management must comprise accurate diagnosis and a careful assessment of the risks attributable to asthma. However, given the widespread availability of effective asthma treatments, the initial focus of assessment has changed from a diagnosis of asthma severity based on symptoms and simple measures of lung function to the achievement of asthma control and an appreciation of those factors that increase the risk of exacerbation. We have therefore further updated the chapter on diagnosis to reflect this significant change in practice, as recommended by international management guidelines.

Once asthma has been diagnosed, successful management is achieved by patients reliably self-managing treatment regimens. Strategies to improve patient self-management and medication use are the best way to achieve best outcomes and quality of life.

Difficult-to-treat asthma is a particular focus of current interest, as the burden of such severe asthma is responsible for the bulk of hospital expenditure in developed countries and considerable impairment of life opportunities in individuals. Recognizing the importance of this and the many different factors contributing to severe asthma, we have expanded the section on refractory asthma, with particular focus on the importance of strategies that assess airway inflammation as a biomarker by which to titrate asthma treatment, since inflammation-guided therapy improves outcomes. As research moves forward, the spectrum of asthma subtypes is increasing, moving us more towards targeted therapy to suit individual patient's needs. Given greater understanding of causal disease pathways, treatments are being expanded to include new therapies that target specific airway inflammatory phenotypes, thus beginning an exciting journey into personalized or stratified medicine for asthma. This development relies on understanding the underlying airway molecular, immunologic and inflammatory pathways responsible for causing different types of asthma and their variable responses to interventions. Recent advances in technology platforms such as genomics, proteomics and metabolomics are helping to expose new causal disease pathways that are likely to lead to important treatment breakthroughs that map onto specific disease subphenotypes.

Overall, the field of asthma remains exciting and is constantly evolving. Our aim with this new edition of *Fast Facts: Asthma* is to incorporate recent trends in an easy-reference format, while not losing sight of new developments, to provide a valuable resource for general practitioners, specialist asthma nurses and others with a keen interest in improving the outcomes of the very many people living with asthma.

Asthma is a chronic inflammatory condition of the airways. It is characterized by recurrent episodes of airflow limitation which, depending on the severity of the attack, produce symptoms such as breathlessness, wheezing, chest tightness and cough. Acute exacerbations can be rapid or gradual in onset, and may be severe and potentially life-threatening.

Autopsy studies of patients who have died from asthma show hyperinflated lungs, with both large and small airways blocked by plugs containing a mixture of mucus, serum proteins, inflammatory cells and cell debris. Microscopic examination reveals extensive inflammatory infiltration of the airways (Figure 1.1), with edema due

Thickened mucosa      Plug of mucus, cells and debris      Thickened sub-basement membrane collagen

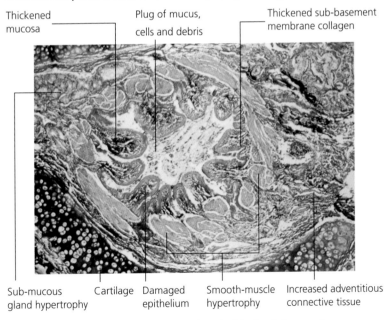

Sub-mucous gland hypertrophy    Cartilage    Damaged epithelium    Smooth-muscle hypertrophy    Increased adventitious connective tissue

**Figure 1.1** Pathological features associated with death from asthma. Airways are blocked by plugs of mucus and inflammatory exudate. There is also vasodilatation and edema, vascular remodeling, smooth muscle hypertrophy and thickening of the basement membrane.

to vasodilatation and blood vessel engorgement, and epithelial disruption. Biopsy studies have shown increased numbers of leukocytes, particularly eosinophils, mast cells and T lymphocytes, in the airways together with increases in the markers of lymphocyte activation. Structural changes resulting from chronic inflammation include bronchial smooth muscle hypertrophy and hyperplasia, new vessel formation, interstitial matrix deposition resulting in basement membrane thickening, and airway wall remodeling.

## Disease mechanisms

In many cases, asthma is an allergic disorder mediated in part by immunoglobulin (Ig)E-dependent mechanisms. Exposure to allergen results in allergen uptake and its presentation by dendritic cells to T helper (Th) lymphocytes (Figure 1.2).

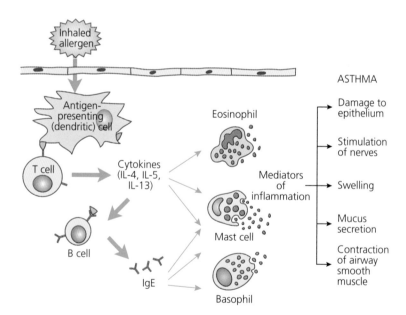

**Figure 1.2** Role of immunoglobulin E (IgE) in airway inflammation and asthma symptoms. Exposure to allergen leads to activation of T lymphocytes, cytokine expression (interleukins [ILs]) and release of IgE from B lymphocytes. IgE binds to cells involved in inflammation, which then release inflammatory mediators.

Th lymphocytes are categorized according to the dominant pattern of cytokines secreted. Those secreting interleukin (IL)-4, IL-5 and IL-13 are Th2, and stimulate the production of IgE from B lymphocytes. Conversely, Th1 lymphocytes produce interferon (IFN)$\gamma$, which facilitates the secretion of IgG by B lymphocytes. T lymphocytes in asthmatic epithelium predominantly release a Th2 pattern of cytokines, indicating the cardinal importance of Th2 lymphocytes in driving the eosinophilic inflammation that is characteristic of asthma.

The IgE produced by the stimulated B lymphocytes binds to mast cells and, possibly, other cells involved in inflammation (e.g. eosinophils), leading to the release of inflammatory mediators. Antigens can also provoke T-cell activation, cytokine and chemokine release, and production of inflammatory mediators. A characteristic finding in asthma, reported only recently, is the presence of mast cells distributed within airway smooth muscle. Moreover, in contrast to the mast cells in the mucosa, which are T-cell-dependent and enriched for the granule enzyme tryptase ($MC_T$), the mast cells in smooth muscle are of the connective-tissue type, enriched in chymase as well as tryptase ($MC_{TC}$). Stimulation of mast cells through IgE-antigen binding or other mechanism results in the release of these mediators together with histamine, and newly generated bronchoconstrictors such as prostaglandin $D_2$ and cysteinyl leukotrienes $LTC_4$ and $LTD_4$. As asthma becomes more severe, the number of $MC_{TC}$ increases in the mucosa at the expense of $MC_T$. This may be important as $MC_{TC}$ are more dependent on stem cell factor (ckit ligand) from mesenchymal and epithelial cells and less responsive to Th2 cytokines and programmed cell death induced by corticosteroids.

**Dysfunction of the airway epithelium.** In addition to immunologic abnormalities leading to asthma, recent findings also point to a fundamental abnormality in asthmatic airway epithelium as a major factor in generating chronic airway inflammation. Dysfunction of the airway epithelial tight junctions leads to greater permeability of the airway surfaces to inhaled particles. These particles can then penetrate the epithelial barrier and elicit inflammatory responses by contact with

9

inflammatory cells such as mast cells and lymphocytes and subepithelial neural pathways.

In addition, the asthmatic epithelium responds to oxidant stress and pathogenic stimulation differently from the non-asthmatic epithelium. Reduced production of the antiviral cytokines IFNβ and IFNλ has been described. This results in impaired clearance of respiratory viruses and, consequently, greater viral replication and persistence during infection of the asthmatic epithelium. This induces inflammation that is more neutrophilic in nature that characterizes asthma exacerbations. It may also, in part, account for the increased morbidity from respiratory viruses in asthma that occurs at certain times of the year, i.e. when respiratory viruses such as those causing the common cold in winter months (e.g. rhinoviruses) are prevalent.

Chronic inflammation is responsible for the two principal manifestations of disordered lung function in asthma: bronchial hyperresponsiveness and acute limitation of airflow (Table 1.1). Patients with asthma show an enhanced airway narrowing (bronchoconstrictor) response to a variety of stimuli such as histamine and methacholine (which act directly on airway smooth muscle), and exercise, hypertonic stimuli (e.g. saline, mannitol), adenosine 5'-monophosphate (AMP) and cold or dry air (which act indirectly), causing bronchoconstriction secondary to the release of inflammatory mediators largely from primed mast cells.

TABLE 1.1

**Manifestations of disordered lung function in asthma**

- Airway hyperresponsiveness
- Variable airflow limitation
  - acute bronchoconstriction
  - swelling of the airway wall
  - chronic mucus plug formation
  - airway wall remodeling
- Stimulation of neurons
  - asthma symptoms

In active asthma, the airway diameter becomes more changeable, as reflected by variation in measures of lung function such as peak expiratory flow (PEF; Figure 1.3). Characteristically in asthma, PEF differs by more than 20% between morning and evening measurements. The mechanisms underlying such diurnal variation in airway caliber are still not known, though the variation is a good marker of poorly controlled asthma.

In asthmatic airways, reductions in airflow can be due to acute bronchoconstriction, swelling of the airway wall, mucous plugging or

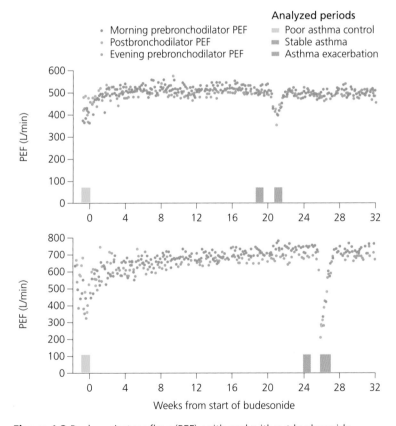

**Figure 1.3** Peak expiratory flow (PEF), with and without budesonide treatment, showing within-day and between-day variations and exacerbations for two patients. Reproduced from Reddel et al. *Lancet* 1999;353:364–9 with permission from Elsevier.

airway wall remodeling. Acute bronchoconstriction may occur as a result of allergen-induced release of inflammatory mediators such as histamine, prostaglandins and leukotrienes. Swelling of the airway wall is caused by edema, with or without bronchoconstriction. Chronic inflammation can also lead to hypersecretion of mucus and exudation, resulting in plugging of the airways and, ultimately, matrix deposition and airway remodeling (see Figure 1.1).

## Definition of asthma based on pathophysiology

An operational definition of asthma in which symptoms are related to the underlying pathophysiology (Table 1.2) has important consequences for diagnosis and treatment. Repeating lung function measurements to take account of the marked variation in airflow in asthma is an important element in the diagnosis (see Chapter 3). Similarly, recognizing that asthma is a chronic inflammatory disorder has focused attention on the use of corticosteroids in long-term management (see Chapter 4).

Historically asthma has been defined as a disease characterized by the presence of eosinophils in mucosal inflammation. Mucosal inflammation can be measured by examination of cell counts in induced sputum (Figure 1.4). Examination of induced sputum cell counts has defined subtypes of asthma based on the presence or

TABLE 1.2

**An operational definition of asthma based on underlying pathophysiology**

- Asthma is a chronic inflammatory disorder of the airways, in which many cells and cellular elements play a role
- The chronic inflammation causes an associated increase in airway hyperresponsiveness that leads to recurrent episodes of wheezing, breathlessness, chest tightness and cough, particularly at night and/or in the early morning
- Episodes of asthma symptoms are usually associated with widespread but variable airflow obstruction that is often reversible, either spontaneously or with treatment

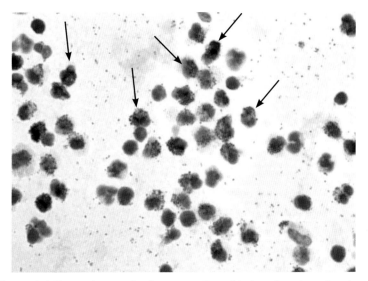

**Figure 1.4** Photomicrograph of a preparation of induced sputum showing eosinophils (arrowed) comprising 46% of cells.

absence of sputum eosinophils. By convention, counts of eosinophils in induced sputum that exceed 3% are associated with significant eosinophilic inflammation. This type of asthma is sometimes referred to as 'Th2 high', as the inflammatory response depends on Th2-type cytokines (IL-3, -4, -5, -9 and -13) as well as chemokines (eotaxin, RANTES). In such patients, the gene profile expressed in epithelial and sputum cells reflects the actions of Th2 cytokines such as IL-4 and IL-13, as well as corticosteroid responsiveness.

However, the inflammatory cell profile in the airways defines other disease subtypes such as neutrophilic and paucigranulocytic (in which there is a normal cellular profile). Such patients tend to express lower levels of epithelial and sputum cell Th2 genes and have fewer corticosteroid-responsive cytokine inflammatory pathways; the non-eosinophilic inflammatory pathways are associated with relative corticosteroid resistance. In individual cases, the definition of the asthmatic inflammatory phenotype is being used to guide therapy and has shown effectiveness in reducing exacerbations. Such stratification of asthma, particularly in those with more severe disease, has implications for targeting therapy to those most responsive.

## Risk factors for asthma

Asthma is a complex condition, and its causes are not fully understood. Risk factors can be categorized as:

- host factors that predispose an individual to asthma
- causal factors, which are environmental factors that influence susceptibility to the development of asthma in predisposed individuals
- trigger factors, which are environmental factors that precipitate asthma exacerbations and/or cause symptoms to persist.

Examples of these factors are shown in Table 1.3. In any given individual, the development of asthma, and the occurrence of acute exacerbations, will be due to an interaction between numerous predisposing, environmental and occupational factors.

**Predisposing factors.** The most important factor predisposing to most asthma is atopy, which is characterized by excessive IgE production in response to common environmental allergens (e.g. from dust mites, animals, pollens and fungi). The prevalence of asthma increases with increasing serum IgE concentration. Up to 80% of children and young adults with asthma are atopic with aeroallergen hypersensitivity dominating. Atopic diseases, including asthma, have strong heritability, accounting for up to 50% of clinical expression.

Childhood asthma is more common in boys than in girls until the age of about 10 years, when the difference disappears. Severe persistent asthma in adults is more frequent in women. There is some evidence that these differences are due to differences in allergen sensitivity and airway responsiveness between the sexes, although the differential effects of hormones and lung growth at puberty may also lead to changes in asthma prevalence.

*Genetics.* Clearly, genetic influences can modify the risk of an individual developing atopy and asthma. While no single gene has been identified as being causative for asthma, several genetic loci have been associated with increased asthma risk, particularly in certain environments resulting in a gene–environment interaction. It is likely that several of these may work synergistically to cause asthma in individuals exposed to appropriate environmental factors. In

TABLE 1.3

**Potential risk factors for the development or exacerbation of asthma**

Predisposing factors
- Genetic predisposition
- Atopy
- Airway hyperresponsiveness
- Sex
- Race/ethnicity
- Family size

Causal factors
- Indoor allergens (domestic mites, animal allergens, cockroach allergen, fungi)
- Outdoor allergens (pollens, fungi)
- Occupational sensitizers
- Tobacco smoking (passive and active)
- Air pollution (outdoor and indoor)
- Respiratory viral infections
- Diet
- Drugs
- Obesity

Trigger factors
- Allergens and drugs
- Pollutants
- Respiratory infections
- Exercise and hyperventilation
- Changes in the weather
- Air pollutants e.g. sulfur dioxide, ozone
- Foods and food additives
- Extreme emotional expression
- Tobacco smoking
- Irritants (e.g. household sprays, paint fumes)

particular, variants of the genes *ADAM33*, *PHF11*, *HLA-G*, *NPSR1* (also known as *GPRA* and *GPR154*), *IRAK3* (also known as *IRAK-M*), *HLA-DQ*, *YKL-40* (also known as *CHI3L1*), *ORMDL3*, *GSDMB*, *SMAD3* and *IL33* are associated with an increased risk of asthma. However, it is important to recognize that each genetic variant contributes only a small amount to the asthma phenotype, with complex gene–gene and gene–environment interactions being involved.

15

*Immune dysregulation.* A rise in the worldwide prevalence of asthma and allergic diseases has been documented in the past three or so decades, particularly in nations that have adopted some aspects of the western lifestyle. This rise has been particularly well described in Eastern European countries where the epidemiological findings of a rise in the prevalence of allergy and asthma have been associated with changes in lifestyle such as newer housing and increasing in-home childcare. However, with recent rapid lifestyle changes being seen in South East Asia and Africa, asthma and associated allergic disease are rapidly increasing in these parts of the world also, particularly in areas of intense urban development.

By contrast, a lower prevalence of asthma has been observed in children raised in rural environments related to animal farming or in anthroposophic lifestyles that restrict the use of antibiotics and antipyretics and promote consumption of fermented vegetables. This suggests that factors such as degree of exposure to microbial products or alterations in gastrointestinal flora may be protective for the development of asthma and atopy. Childhood infections such as tuberculosis, *Helicobacter pylori* infection and hepatitis are also linked to reduced allergy and asthma, but the effects may be indirect.

Co-incident with the increase of asthma and allergic diseases is the increase in other autoimmune diseases such as juvenile diabetes mellitus, Crohn's disease and juvenile arthritis. These findings are sometimes referred to as the 'hygiene hypothesis', which attributes the rising prevalence of asthma and allergic diseases to a failure in immune maturation caused by the relative protection from bacterial infection and changed gut bacterial flora in the first few years of life that are associated with a western lifestyle. Lack of bacterial stimulation of the immature immune system leads to impaired production of regulatory T-cells and enhancement of Th2 and Th1 responses causatively linked to allergy and autoimmune disease, respectively.

Further understanding of immune maturation is necessary before the networks involved can be fully traced, but the hypothesis has led to trials of bacterial products such as probiotics as potential protective agents for the development of asthma and allergies. Such studies have so far not delivered on their initial promise.

*Nutrition.* Dietary factors have been associated with asthma and allergic disease. In particular, lower levels of vitamin D have been associated with an increased prevalence of asthma and allergic disease in ecologic studies comparing disease rates in temperate and tropical environments. Trials of dietary intervention with supplements are currently under way.

**Causal factors.** The relevance of different causes of asthma depends on individual exposure and when it occurs. In early childhood, inhaled allergens and infection appear to be important causal factors for asthma. In adults, cigarette smoking and exposure to occupational allergens are more likely to be important causal factors.

*Inhaled allergens.* Common indoor sources of inhaled allergens include domestic mites, cats, dogs and fungi. Outdoor pollens from grasses, trees and wind-pollinated weeds are also common inhaled allergens. Allergen exposure leads to the activation of specific T lymphocytes and the production of specific IgE by B lymphocytes, which sensitizes the individual to subsequent exposure. There is a strong correlation between the prevalence of asthma and long-term exposure to allergen, and asthma often improves when the allergen is removed, although this is not always feasible.

Domestic mites appear to be the most common sources of indoor allergens. The principal species involved are *Dermatophagoides pteronyssinus*, *D. farinae*, *D. microceras* and *Euroglyphus mainei*; these account for about 90% of mites in house dust in temperate climates. The predominant allergens are amylase, and cysteine and serine proteases from the digestive tracts of the mites and their feces. In inner cities and tropical environments, cockroaches are also a source of inhalant allergens.

Domestic animals release allergens in their saliva, urine, feces and danders. The most important allergen is the Fel d 1 allergen found in cat fur and saliva. Allergic sensitivity to dogs is less common but, nevertheless, up to 30% of allergic patients have positive skin tests to dog allergens. Other domestic pets, particularly horses, rabbits, guinea pigs, rats, gerbils and mice, are also important sources of sensitizing allergen.

Both indoor and outdoor fungi can act as allergens. The most important fungi to have been associated with asthma are *Aspergillus* and *Alternaria*. Chronic colonization of the airways with *Aspergillus* can be associated with severe asthma, particularly in those who are also allergic to this mold. Pollen allergens associated with asthma are derived from trees (predominantly in early spring), grasses (late spring and summer) and weeds (late summer and autumn).

*Occupation-related factors* are summarized in Table 1.4. High-molecular-weight sensitizers such as grain, dust, urine and dander proteins from animals probably cause sensitization by the same IgE-dependent mechanisms as allergens. The mechanisms through which low-molecular-weight sensitizers (such as di-isocyanates and platinum salts) act is unknown; however, in some cases, there is increasing evidence that IgE plays a role.

*Drugs.* Among the most common causes of drug-induced asthma are acetylsalicylic acid (ASA; aspirin) and other non-steroidal anti-inflammatory drugs (NSAIDs), which have been described as triggering asthma attacks in 4–28% of asthmatic patients. Intolerance to NSAIDs usually develops between 30 and 50 years of age, and persists throughout life. It results from a defect in the oxidative metabolism of arachidonic acid, causing excessive production of a powerful class of cysteinyl leukotrienes. Individuals with NSAID-hypersensitive asthma commonly have nasal polyposis and typically have florid eosinophilic asthma despite often being non-atopic. Exposure to acetaminophen (paracetamol) early in life has also been linked to asthma.

*Exposure to cigarette smoke* is one of the potentially modifiable causes of asthma. Passive exposure is an important early-life risk factor for asthma, impairing lung growth and encouraging allergic responses in early infancy. Children exposed to cigarette smoke, especially from their mothers, have a significantly increased risk of asthma and exacerbations. In adults, there is some evidence that smoking may increase the risk of developing asthma after exposure to some occupational sensitizers. In addition, current smoking is associated with an increase in symptoms and blunted response to preventive treatments, especially steroids.

TABLE 1.4

**Some causes of occupational asthma**

| Occupation/<br>occupational field | Agent |
| --- | --- |
| | **Animal proteins** |
| Laboratory animal workers, vet | Dander and urine proteins |
| Food processing | Shellfish, egg proteins, pancreatic enzymes, amylase |
| Dairy farmers | Storage mites |
| Poultry farmers | Poultry mites, droppings, feathers |
| Granary workers | Storage mites, *Aspergillus* spp., indoor ragweed, grass |
| Research workers | Locusts, animal allergens |
| Fish-food manufacturing | Midges |
| Detergent manufacturing | *Bacillus subtilis* enzymes |
| Silk workers | Silkworm moths and larvae |
| | **Plant proteins** |
| Bakers | Flour, amylase |
| Food processing | Coffee-bean dust, meat tenderizer (papain), tea |
| Farmers | Soybean dust |
| Shipping workers | Grain dust (mold, insects, grain) |
| Laxative manufacturing | Ispaghula, psyllium |
| Sawmill workers, carpenters | Wood dust (western red cedar, oak, mahogany, zebrawood, redwood, Lebanon cedar, African maple, eastern white cedar) |
| Electric soldering | Colophony (pine resin) |
| Nurses | Psyllium, latex |

CONTINUED

TABLE 1.4 (CONTINUED)

| Occupation/ occupational field | Agent |
| --- | --- |
| **Inorganic chemicals** | |
| Refinery workers | Platinum salts, vanadium salts |
| Plating | |
| Diamond polishing | Cobalt salts |
| Manufacturing | Aluminum fluoride |
| Beauticians | Persulfate, latex |
| Welding | Stainless-steel fumes, chromium salts |
| **Organic chemicals** | |
| Manufacturing | |
| Hospital workers | Disinfectants (sulfathiazole, chloramines, formaldehyde, glutaraldehyde), latex |
| Anesthesiology | Enflurane |
| Fur dyeing | Fur dye |
| Rubber processing | Formaldehyde, ethylene diamine, phthalic anhydride, triethylene tetramines, trimellitic anhydride, hexamethyl tetramine, acrylates |
| Automobile painting | Ethanolamine, diisocyanates |
| Foundry workers | Reaction product of furan binder |

*Pollution.* Laboratory studies have identified a number of air pollutants as factors in worsening asthma, but epidemiological studies of the relationship between outdoor air pollution and asthma have yielded conflicting results. Although asthma is more common in industrialized countries (see Chapter 2), there is little evidence that air pollution alone is directly responsible for this increase in prevalence; in some, such as China, India and Japan, it may contribute. Importantly, indoor pollutants arising from, for example, heating and cooking with gas or on wood fires, and organic chemicals used in buildings and furnishings appear to be associated with increases in prevalence in some instances. Exposure to air pollution, especially that associated with summer episodes (e.g. ozone), is a well-established cause of exacerbations of established asthma.

*Diet.* The relationship between asthma and dietary factors is unclear. There is some evidence that asthma is associated with food allergy during infancy, which often precedes other atopic disorders such as allergic rhinitis and, frequently, asthma. Trials of dietary modification in which highly 'allergenic' foods have been avoided in pregnancy and the first year of life have shown some benefit in delaying the onset of allergic eczema, but not in reducing the eventual occurrence of asthma. Widespread recommendations to reduce intake of allergenic foods early in life have not resulted in a reduction in food sensitivity. Indeed, some evidence from animal studies suggests that early introduction of solids may protect from food allergies. Therefore, dietary modifications during pregnancy and infancy to prevent asthma are not currently recommended as isolated interventions. Babies should be breastfed for at least 6 months. There is some evidence that this, combined with a low-allergen environment and reduced exposure to dust mites and household pets, is helpful, but delayed introduction of foods is not recommended.

Epidemiological evidence suggests that diets high in omega-3 fatty acids (mainly acquired from fish oils) may be protective against asthma, as well as diets high in fruit and vegetables rich in antioxidants.

*Infections.* Respiratory viral infections are well established as a cause of asthma exacerbations; they have been detected in over 80% of children with an exacerbation. The role of particular infections, such as rhinoviruses, as a cause of asthma in early life, is becoming increasingly well established, particularly in association with allergen exposure. Reduced antiviral innate immunity (reduced IFN induction) that leads to frequent wheezing in infancy is a powerful predictor of asthma by age 6 years and, in parallel, also predisposes to allergen sensitization. This has been named the 'two hit hypothesis' for the origins of asthma.

*Obesity* is considered a major risk factor for asthma. Obesity-induced changes in hormone metabolism and production of adipokines by adipose tissue may lead to a low-grade systemic inflammation that involves the lung. In addition, some of the comorbidities of obesity, such as reduced ventilatory capacity, gastroesophageal reflux and sleep-disordered breathing, may trigger asthma or asthma-like symptoms.

**Trigger factors** can induce asthma by causing inflammation, provoking bronchial hyperresponsive airways to contract or both. Individual triggers vary markedly, and may alter with time in the same patient. Common triggers include allergens, air pollutants, viral infections, exercise and hyperventilation, and emotional stress. Adverse weather conditions have been associated with asthma exacerbations, particularly following thunderstorms, when there is osmotic release of allergen nanoparticles from pollen grains.

## Key points – pathophysiology

- Asthma is a chronic inflammatory condition of the conducting airways. It is characterized by recurrent episodes of airflow limitation which, depending on the severity of the attack, can cause breathlessness, wheezing, chest tightness, cough and, rarely, death
- Structural changes also occur in the airways; these are particularly evident in those with severe and chronic asthma.
- The structural abnormalities in asthma include thickened basement membrane, mucus hypersecretion, smooth muscle hypertrophy, and mast cells within the airway smooth muscle.
- Airway inflammation in people with asthma is not uniform: in most it is eosinophil predominant, but in others neutrophil cell types predominate.
- The most prominent risk factors are allergen exposure in genetically susceptible individuals and maternal cigarette smoking.
- Genetic factors determine susceptibility to environmental factors, and it is the interaction between these that leads to clinical disease.

## Key references

Anderson GP. Endotyping asthma: new insights into key pathogenic mechanisms in a complex, heterogeneous disease. *Lancet* 2008;372:1107–19.

Arshad SH. Primary prevention of asthma and allergy. *J Allergy Clin Immunol* 2005;116:3–14.

Brightling CE, Bradding P, Symon FA et al. Mast-cell infiltration of airway smooth muscle in asthma. *N Engl J Med* 2002;346:1699–705.

Haldar P, Pavord ID, Shaw DE et al. Cluster analysis and clinical asthma phenotypes. *Am J Respir Crit Care Med* 2008;178:218–24.

Holgate ST. Epithelium dysfunction in asthma. *J Allergy Clin Immunol* 2007;120:1233–44.

Moffatt MF, Gut IG, Demenais F et al. A large-scale, consortium-based genomewide association study of asthma. *N Engl J Med* 2010;363:1211–21.

Schaub B, Lauener R, von Mutius E. The many faces of the hygiene hypothesis. *J Allergy Clin Immunol* 2006;117:969–77.

Shore SA. Obesity and asthma: possible mechanisms. *J Allergy Clin Immunol* 2008;121:1087–93.

Asthma is one of the most common chronic diseases worldwide. The reported prevalence depends on the definition of asthma used, whether relying on self-report of symptoms, or whether these are further validated by lung function testing or doctor diagnosis. The prevalence of asthma also depends on the age, geographic region and socioeconomic status of the population studied, and the study design. Several large international trials have studied asthma prevalence in adults and children.

## Prevalence

**Childhood.** The International Study of Asthma and Allergies in Childhood (ISAAC) has provided cross-sectional data from many global sites since 1993, with the most recent survey in 2003. In this study, the prevalence of asthma in populations of children aged 13–14 years and 6–7 years is, on average, 13.7% and 11.6%, respectively. However, in some nations, particularly in high-income countries, prevalence in the 13–14 years age group exceeds 20%, indicating very large regional differences in asthma prevalence (Figure 2.1). Studies have consistently shown that the prevalence of asthma increased worldwide through the 1980s and 1990s. However, in countries with a very high prevalence of asthma historically, particularly English-speaking countries, the rates have stabilized or are even falling. In contrast, the prevalence in developing countries appears to be increasing, particularly in some parts of Asia, Africa and South America.

**Adulthood.** The prevalence of asthma in adults has not been the subject of such widespread global initiatives as the investigation of asthma in children. What evidence there is has been drawn from studies of younger adults (Figure 2.2), to avoid confusion with other diseases occurring later in life such as chronic obstructive pulmonary disease. The European Community Respiratory Health Survey has established

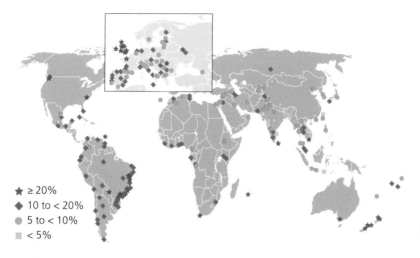

★ ≥ 20%
◆ 10 to < 20%
● 5 to < 10%
▪ < 5%

The ★ shows the centers reporting the highest prevalence

**Figure 2.1** The prevalence of asthma in 13–14 year olds reported by centers around the world. While high-income countries report high prevalence of asthma, there is over a 15-fold variation of asthma symptom prevalence between countries; middle- and low-income nations also report high asthma prevalence. Data were collected by the International Study of Allergies and Asthma in Childhood (ISAAC) from 1993 to 2003. Note that while asthma prevalence in this age group has usually stabilized or declined in high-income countries, asthma prevalence continues to increase in low-income countries, with a high proportion of those with asthma suffering severe symptoms. Source: The International Union Against Tuberculosis and Lung Disease, 2011.

that the prevalence of wheeze consistent with asthma ranges from 4.1 to 32%, with a median of 20.7%. However, symptoms of wheeze occur with greater prevalence than airway hyperresponsiveness, which range from 3.4 to 28% with a median of 13%.

Within a particular country, the prevalence of asthma may differ markedly between different racial and ethnic groups. For example, in the USA asthma is more common among black African–Americans than whites, but the difference is less pronounced in the UK. In the UK, the prevalence of asthma among Asians is lower than among

25

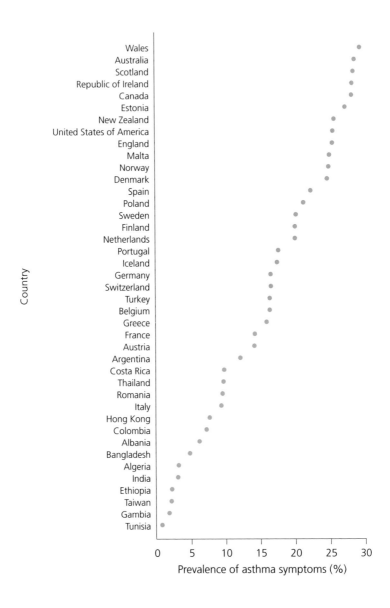

**Figure 2.2** The prevalence of asthma according to questionnaire in adults aged 20 to 44 years. Prevalence rates of self-reported wheezing range from 1 to 30%. Reproduced from Masoli et al. 2004, with permission from the Global Initiative for Asthma.

whites, although this trend may be changing with the adoption of domestic lifestyle changes.

Asthma appears to be more prevalent in urbanized countries; the reasons are not clear, but may include:

- exposure to domestic allergens, particularly house dust mites and cockroach
- exposure to occupational allergens
- increased urbanization and thus exposure to adjuvants such as respiratory viruses, dietary components and petrochemical pollutants
- reduced exposure to bacterial and viral infections in early infancy.

## Mortality

Death rates from asthma are usually reported for the under 35s, as the report of an asthma-related death in this age group is relatively reliable (Figure 2.3). In older age groups the reported mortality from asthma can be inflated because of comorbidities, such as COPD. Wide variation in case–fatality rates is seen worldwide (Figure 2.4), which may reflect differences in both the availability and the delivery of effective asthma care and medication to individuals with symptomatic asthma.

Asthma death rates not only vary between nations but have also fluctuated over time. In many countries, a marked increase in asthma deaths occurred in the 1960s, after which mortality decreased. In the UK, the mortality rate increased slightly during the 1980s, but the most recent data indicate that death rates are now falling. The greatest increase in mortality during the late 1970s and 1980s was seen in New Zealand (Figure 2.5). The reasons for this are unclear; the use of high doses of short-acting $\beta_2$-agonists (SABAs), especially high-dose fenoterolin, has been associated with the increased mortality, but the evidence is inconclusive. Ethnic and socioeconomic factors may be at least partly responsible. In New Zealand, a large proportion of the increased mortality occurred in Maoris, and during the same period a similar increase occurred among black Americans living in inner-city areas of the USA. Studies of asthma deaths during this time suggested that a majority were preventable with the best available current

27

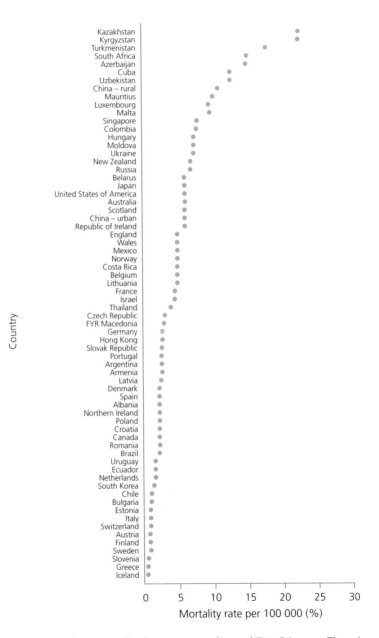

**Figure 2.3** Asthma mortality in young people aged 5 to 34 years. There is substantial regional variation. Reproduced from Masoli et al. 2004, with permission from the Global Initiative for Asthma.

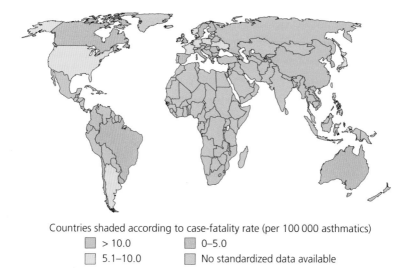

Countries shaded according to case-fatality rate (per 100 000 asthmatics)
- [ ] > 10.0
- [ ] 5.1–10.0
- [ ] 0–5.0
- [ ] No standardized data available

**Figure 2.4** Asthma mortality rates in individual countries where data are available, adjusted for the asthma prevalence in that nation. The substantial variation suggests that access to treatment and other preventive measures are likely to influence asthma mortality rates. Reproduced from Masoli et al. 2004, with permission from the Global Initiative for Asthma.

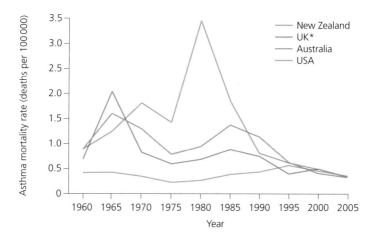

**Figure 2.5** Asthma mortality rate (deaths per 100 000) in people aged 5–34 years in Australia, New Zealand, the UK and the USA betwen 1960 and 2005. *Data for England and Wales only 1960–1995. Adapted from data in Wijesinghe et al., 2009

treatment, and that factors such as poor access to healthcare may
have been partly responsible. In countries that have introduced effective
guidelines for asthma management (e.g. UK, Australia and Scandinavian
countries), mortality has declined and is now reasonably stable.

Asthma in older people has also become a recent focus of attention.
With the gradual reduction in asthma mortality in younger age
groups, people over the age of 55 years are now the group who most
commonly die of asthma – particularly in higher income nations. In
this group, there is uncertainty as to a correct diagnosis of asthma or
COPD; further research will be required to determine the extent of
asthma in older people and effective therapies for this group.

## Morbidity

In addition to being an important cause of death, asthma causes
substantial morbidity and interference with everyday activities.
Insights into the extent of asthma-related morbidity come from
surveys examining the severity of asthma symptoms. Surveys
conducted by telephone across Europe, the USA and the Asia Pacific
region reveal that while the severity of symptoms varies between
regions, severe asthma symptoms – including nightly waking with
asthma and asthma symptoms more than twice daily – are present in
between 11% and 32% of those surveyed (Figure 2.6). This study also
revealed that in every region, around 30% of individuals with asthma
presented for emergency medical care for their asthma annually.

Further evidence of the morbidity of asthma comes from studies
of hospital admissions for asthma. These show marked geographical
variations in large part influenced both by asthma prevalence and the
healthcare delivery system in place. Since asthma exacerbations
resulting in emergency medical attendances and hospital admission as
well as symptoms are usually able to be prevented and controlled with
medications, this variation suggests a lack of use or availability of
known effective anti-asthma medications.

Increasing morbidity may relate to a number of factors, including:
• the increasing prevalence of asthma
• increased exposure to trigger factors (e.g. allergens, pollutants,
viruses)

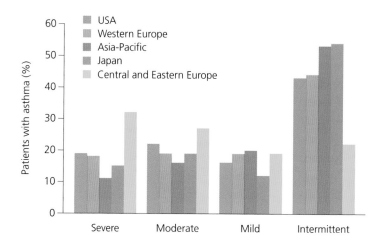

**Figure 2.6** Asthma symptom severity among asthma patients from five regions. Adapted from data in Rabe et al., 2004.

- undertreatment with, or reduced access to, anti-inflammatory agents
- overdependence on bronchodilators
- failure to monitor lung function by regular peak expiratory flow (PEF) measurements or spirometry
- health economic factors
- poor coordination of care pathways e.g. overdependence on the hospital sector.

## Early-life origins of asthma

Studies in neonates and young children born of allergic parents suggest that the atopic state begins to manifest itself very early in life. Thus, the findings of increased numbers of mast cells and eosinophils in the lavage fluid of children with asthma aged 3–5 years suggest that all the necessary cell and mediator pathways are already in place to express the full disease. Despite several recent large intervention studies, such as the Childhood Asthma Management Program (CAMP) and START (Inhaled Steroid Treatment as Regular Therapy in Early Asthma), it is still not clear that early introduction of inhaled corticosteroids at the

31

onset of asthma influences the natural history of the disease or airway remodeling. Recent studies suggest that it does not.

There may be maternal risk factors that influence the genetic expression of allergy and asthma in the offspring. Several laboratories have now shown that lymphocytes from the cord blood of babies of allergic mothers show delayed maturation, particularly in respect of the cytokine interferon-γ, which, under normal conditions, has the capacity to inhibit the development of the allergic pathways. The basis for this deficiency is far from clear, but it does provide one potential avenue for correcting an immunologic response early in life before the allergic cells are recruited into the lung. This T cell defect in the origins of asthma also aligns with the deficiency of primary interferons in the epithelium in response to viral infections and increased risk of atopic sensitization.

## Natural history of asthma

Asthma can occur at any time in life, although it most commonly develops in infancy and childhood. The natural history of the condition varies according to the age at onset, and possibly according to the causative factors.

**Infancy (0–3 years).** Wheezing is common in the early years of life and recent studies have enabled the identification of several distinct phenotypes. The most common are:

- transient infantile wheeze, in which children have recurrent wheeze during the first few years of life, but rarely thereafter
- episodic wheeze, where children have wheeze associated with viral infections that does not persist between attacks
- atopic asthma, in which children are usually allergic and often have other allergic diseases such as allergic rhinitis and eczema.

Atopic asthma is generally more likely to persist into childhood than the other wheezing phenotypes, whilst episodic wheezing may resolve later in childhood.

**Childhood.** Allergy, particularly to house-dust mites, is the most common feature associated with the development of asthma during childhood. Viral infections are important triggers of exacerbations in children with atopic asthma and may cooperate with allergen sensitization in the origins of asthma. By the age of 8 years, a significant proportion of children develop bronchial hyperresponsiveness and symptoms of moderate-to-severe asthma, whereas others continue to show mild intermittent asthma. These different natural histories of the disease over the life course suggest different phenotypes and engagement of different causative pathways.

Lung growth is relatively normal in most children with mild asthma, but may be reduced in children with severe persistent symptoms. This is important – long-term studies show that, although asthma disappears in 30–50% of children during puberty, it often recurs in adulthood. Furthermore, lung function often remains impaired even when clinical signs of asthma have disappeared, and 5–10% of children with mild asthma develop severe asthma later in life. In general, children with mild asthma are likely to have a good prognosis, but those with moderate or severe asthma are more likely to show some degree of bronchial hyperresponsiveness and to be at risk for the persistence of asthma and progressive decline in lung function throughout life.

Although counterintuitive based on the inflammatory concept of asthma, there is no evidence that regular use of powerful inhaled corticosteroids in early life alters the natural history of asthma even though these drugs are highly effective in disease control, and reduce the burden of symptoms and exacerbations. There is evidence that eczema is a major risk for the persistence of childhood asthma into adult life. As both diseases have defects in barrier function, a causative link is implied, possibly through an enhanced opportunity for allergens to penetrate and sensitize.

Prevalence studies reveal that asthma is generally more common in boys until puberty, when more girls develop asthma and the predominance reverses. Some individuals acquire asthma in their adolescent years. As the prevalence of asthma in adults is generally lower than in children, it is evident that many children grow out of childhood asthma. Cohort studies following children to age 40 years reveal that approximately two-thirds of those with asthma at age

7 years did not have current asthma by the age of 40, with a slightly higher number of men undergoing remission than women. Those whose asthma remits tend to have less severe and persistent asthma in childhood. Asthma acquired in childhood is more likely to remit than asthma acquired in either adolescence or adulthood.

**Adulthood.** The development of asthma in adulthood is frequently associated with exposure to occupational sensitizers, causing classic allergic responses, or via mechanisms not involving atopy. It is not known what proportion of patients who develop asthma in adulthood actually had a history of childhood asthma – abnormal lung function or bronchial hyperresponsiveness persists in many patients whose symptoms disappear during childhood. Indeed there is increasing evidence that what may be considered as late-onset asthma may well have started in childhood, remitted and then returned. However, for late-onset non-atopic asthma, the etiology is likely to be different.

The natural history of late-onset asthma is variable. It appears that lung function (as measured by the forced expiratory volume in 1 second [$FEV_1$]) deteriorates at a faster rate in patients whose asthma develops after the age of about 50 years than in those who develop asthma at an earlier age. Moreover, bronchial hyperresponsiveness appears to be associated with an accelerated rate of deterioration. Such older people with asthma have increasingly become the focus of attention as the mortality and symptom burden of this group is high and response to controller therapy more variable.

## Key points – epidemiology and natural history

- Asthma is one of the most common chronic diseases worldwide. The highest prevalence is seen in affluent westernized populations.
- In many countries asthma, along with other allergic disorders, continues to increase in prevalence, especially in children and young adults.
- Death from asthma reflects poor access to healthcare in many countries.
- Asthma can occur at any time in life, although it most commonly develops in infancy and childhood.
- There is evidence that early life events, including those that occur in the womb, may be important in the initiation of childhood asthma in those genetically at risk.
- Although asthma disappears in 30–50% of children during puberty, it often recurs in adulthood.
- There is no evidence that regular use of corticosteroids in early life alters the natural history of asthma, though these medications are highly effective in disease control.

## Key references

Asher MI, Montefort S, Björkstén B et al. Worldwide time trends in the prevalence of symptoms of asthma, allergic rhinoconjunctivitis, and eczema in childhood: ISAAC Phases One and Three repeat multicountry cross-sectional surveys. *Lancet* 2006;368:733–43.

Burgess JA, Matheson MC, Gurrin LC et al. Factors influencing asthma remission: a longitudinal study from childhood to middle age. *Thorax* 2011;66:508–13.

The Childhood Asthma Management Program Research Group. Long-term effects of budesonide or nedocromil in children with asthma. *N Engl J Med* 2000;343:1054–63.

Holt PG, Upham JW, Sly PD. Contemporaneous maturation of immunologic and respiratory functions during early childhood: implications for development of asthma prevention strategies. *J Allergy Clin Immunol* 2005;116: 16–24.

The International Union Against Tuberculosis and Lung Disease. *The Global Asthma Report 2011*. Paris: The International Union Against Tuberculosis and Lung Disease, 2011. Available from www.theunion. org/images/stories/pressrelease/ Global_asthma-report.pdf, last accessed 12 March 2013.

Masoli M, Fabian D, Holt S, Beasley R. *Global Burden of Asthma*. Report developed for the Global Initiative for Asthma, 2004. Available from www.ginasthma.org/ pdf/GINABurdenReport.pdf, last accessed 12 March 2013.

Pauwels RA, Pedersen S, Busse WW et al. Early intervention with budesonide in mild persistent asthma: a randomised, double-blind trial. *Lancet* 2003;361:1071–6.

Rabe KF, Adachi M, Lai CKW et al. Worldwide severity and control of asthma in children and adults: The global Asthma Insights and Reality surveys. *J Allergy Clin Immunol* 2004:114:40–7.

Sly PD, Boner AL, Björksten B et al. Early identification of atopy in the prediction of persistent asthma in children. *Lancet* 2008;372:1100–6.

Wijesinghe M, Weatherall M, Perrin K et al. International trends in asthma mortality rates in the 5- to 34-year age group: a call for closer surveillance. *Chest* 2009;135: 1045–9.

# 3  Diagnosis and classification

Although asthma is one of the most common chronic disorders it is often underdiagnosed, especially in older people. Because of the intermittent and non-specific nature of symptoms, patients may accept the effects of their condition and delay seeking treatment. They may also be incorrectly diagnosed when they do seek medical advice: asthma is often misdiagnosed as bronchitis or 'wheezy' bronchitis, particularly in children and the elderly, and is treated inappropriately with antibiotics. An accurate diagnosis is essential for effective asthma control.

## Symptoms

The clinical diagnosis of asthma is often based on the presence of symptoms such as:

- breathlessness – often episodic
- wheeze
- chest tightness
- cough.

These symptoms may be particularly marked at night and in the early hours of the morning. The presence of symptoms, however, is not by itself sufficient for a diagnosis of asthma; the history of symptoms and possible provocative factors must also be considered (Table 3.1), and the diagnosis confirmed by objective measures of lung function. Various symptom scoring scales have been developed to monitor the occurrence and severity of symptoms. These can be useful in the management of individual patients, although it is important that they be adapted according to the patient's age and cultural background.

## Physical examination

Asthma symptoms vary during the day, and the respiratory system may appear normal on physical examination. During asthma exacerbations, small airways are occluded through a combination of bronchoconstriction, edema and hypersecretion of mucus. The patient

TABLE 3.1

**Key questions to consider in making a diagnosis of asthma**

Consider asthma if the answer to any of the following is 'yes'

- Has the patient had an attack or recurrent episodes of wheezing?
- Does the patient have a troublesome cough, particularly at night or on waking?
- Is the patient awoken by coughing or difficulty in breathing?
- Does the patient cough or wheeze after physical activity?
- Does the patient experience breathing difficulties during a particular season?
- Does the patient cough, wheeze or develop chest tightness after exposure to airborne allergens or irritants?
- Do colds go to the chest or take more than 10 days to resolve?
- Does the patient use any medication when symptoms occur? If so, how often?
- Are symptoms relieved when medication is used?

therefore breathes at a higher lung volume to maintain airway patency. Consequently, clinical signs of dyspnea (Table 3.2) are more likely to be present during symptomatic exacerbations or if patients are examined in the morning before administration of a bronchodilator.

The absence of wheezing is not sufficient to preclude a diagnosis of asthma. In an exacerbation, some patients may have such severe obstruction of the airways that wheezing may not be noticeable. Such patients usually have other signs of respiratory obstruction, such as difficulty in speaking, cyanosis, drowsiness and chest hyperinflation.

## Measurements of lung function

Patients with asthma often have poor recognition of their symptoms and poor perception of symptom severity. Measurements of lung function provide an objective assessment of airflow limitation, and its variability and reversibility, and thus are valuable in the diagnosis and management of asthma. Measurements widely used in patients over

TABLE 3.2

**Clinical signs of asthma**

- Dyspnea
    - wheezing, particularly on expiration
    - use of the accessory muscles of respiration
    - flaring of the nostrils during inspiration (particularly in children)
    - interrupted talking
    - hyperinflation (use of accessory muscles, hunched shoulders, hunching forward or preferring not to lie down)
- Cough
    - chronic or recurring
    - worse at night and in the early hours of the morning; sleep disrupted
- Tachycardia
- Associated conditions
    - eczema
    - rhinitis
    - sinusitis
    - hay fever
- Cyanosis – life-threatening!
- Drowsiness – life-threatening!

5 years of age are forced expiratory volume in 1 second ($FEV_1$), forced vital capacity (FVC) and peak expiratory flow (PEF).

$FEV_1$ and FVC are measured by spirometry (Figure 3.1), although electronic portable devices are becoming increasingly available. To make these measurements, patients are taught to perform a forced expiration after a maximal inspiration, and the highest of at least three reproducible measurements is recorded. Predicted values based on age, sex, race and height are available and can be compared with the patient's measurements to aid interpretation. The ratio of $FEV_1$ to FVC provides a useful measure of airway obstruction. Forced expiration normally produces $FEV_1$/FVC ratios of more than 70%

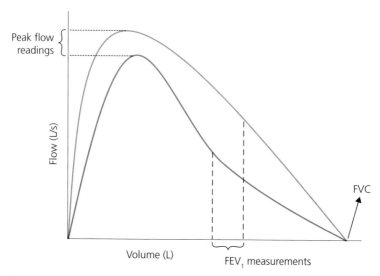

Peak flow readings

Flow (L/s)

FVC

Volume (L)

$FEV_1$ measurements

**Figure 3.1** Flow volume loop (spirometry) showing a trace of flow versus volume in maximal exhalation pre- (red line) and post (blue line) bronchodilator medication. Peak flow and $FEV_1$ are extrapolated from this curve. Both peak flow and $FEV_1$ post-bronchodilator are greater than their pre-bronchodilator measurements, typical of asthma. FVC, forced vital capacity.

(or 85% in children); ratios below these figures suggest airway obstruction: the lower the ratio, the more severe the obstruction.

Spirometers have become much smaller and more portable; while spirometry is usually carried out in the hospital or specialist setting, it is increasingly available in an office setting, such as a general practice room. If spirometry is used to monitor patients, it is critical that the tester is appropriately trained in conducting the test and in maintaining the equipment to ensure reproducibility and comparability of measurements.

For asthma diagnosis, spirometry is usually assessed before and after the administration of an inhaled short-acting $\beta_2$-agonist (SABA): responsiveness of $FEV_1$ by 12% or 200 mL (whichever is the greater) is indicative of asthma. Measurement of PEF by means of a peak flow meter provides a useful and practical alternative to spirometry. In most patients, there is a good correlation between PEF and $FEV_1$.

Peak flow meters are small, convenient, inexpensive and suitable for home use. They can be used both for the diagnosis of asthma in the clinic (Table 3.3) and to monitor asthma in the home. Changes in PEF can precede the onset of symptoms during acute exacerbations in some individuals; thus, early detection of such changes can allow appropriate treatment to be given. PEF readings can also indicate to an individual the severity of their asthma when compared with previous readings, enabling institution of a self-management plan.

Several types of peak flow meter are available, but the basic technique for use is the same in each case (Figure 3.2). Ideally, patients should measure PEF immediately on waking before taking any bronchodilator medication and last thing at night after taking bronchodilator. Variability in daily PEF can then be calculated as a percentage of the mean daily value:

$$\text{Daily variability (\%)} = \frac{PEF_{evening} - PEF_{morning}}{1/2\ (PEF_{evening} + PEF_{morning})} \times 100$$

Daily variability of more than 20% indicates asthma.

TABLE 3.3

**Diagnosis of asthma from peak expiratory flow (PEF) measurements**

- PEF increases by more than 15% and at least 60 L/min 15–20 minutes after inhalation of a short-acting $\beta_2$-agonist (e.g. salbutamol or terbutaline)
- PEF varies by more than 20% between morning measurement on waking and measurement 12 hours later
- PEF decreases by more than 15% after 6 minutes of running or other exercise

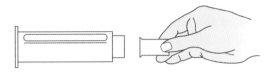

Put the disposable
mouthpiece on the
peak flow meter.

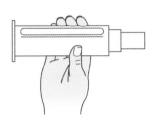

Stand up and hold
the peak flow meter
horizontally. Make sure
that the end of the
marker is at the end of
the scale and that your
hand is not restricting
marker movement.

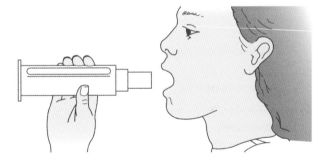

Breathe in
as deeply
as you can.

Then close your lips
tightly around the
mouthpiece and
breathe out quickly.
Note the results and
repeat the procedure
twice. Use the highest
reading.

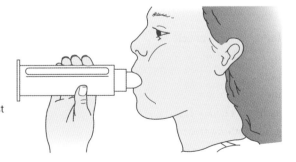

**Figure 3.2** Use of a peak flow meter.

## Measurement of bronchial responsiveness

Measurement of bronchial responsiveness can be useful in the diagnosis of asthma, although there is some overlap between the range of values found in patients with asthma and in those with rhinitis or other causes of lower airway obstruction, such as chronic obstructive pulmonary disease (COPD).

The most usual tests are performed in a lung function laboratory and involve the patient inhaling incremental doses of a bronchoconstricting substance, such as histamine, methacholine, hypertonic saline, adenosine 5'-monophosphate (AMP) or mannitol. Tests using the last three measure 'indirect' bronchial responsiveness and take into account the inflammatory cell priming that is a crucial component of the disease. These tests are said to be more specific as diagnostic tools. Whichever agonist is applied, spirometry is used to follow the changes in airway caliber. Airway responsiveness is usually defined as that dose (D) or concentration (C) of the agonist that reduces the $FEV_1$ by 20% of the starting volume (i.e. PD20 or PC20). A standardized exercise test has also found use, especially in young children with suspected asthma.

## Measurement of airway inflammation

Asthma can also be classified according to the inflammation found in the airways. While asthma has been characteristically associated with eosinophilic airway inflammation, the presence of non-eosinophilic inflammation may suggest types of asthma that are more likely to be corticosteroid refractory.

**Induced sputum cellularity.** Airway inflammation is usually detected by examination of induced sputum cellularity (see Figure 1.4). The presence of eosinophils at greater than 3% of non-squamous cells is indicative of eosinophilic inflammation in the airways and 'Th2-high' asthma. The analysis of sputum inflammatory cells has been used to guide asthma treatment, with reports indicating treatment guided by sputum eosinophil counts is effective in reducing the rate of asthma exacerbations. Low levels of eosinophils represent the 'Th2 low' phenotype that is less responsive to corticosteroids.

43

**Nitric oxide in exhaled air.** The concentration of nitric oxide (NO) in exhaled air can be used as a surrogate measure for airway inflammation in asthma. NO is released from the airway epithelium. It increases in inflammatory disorders, and high levels are a feature of 'Th2-high' or eosinophilic airway inflammation.

It is measured using specific equipment, some of which is portable and therefore may provide a useful point-of-care test. Since the concentration of exhaled NO varies with the expiratory flow rate, values are generated at a standardized 50 mL/s, a submaximal expiratory flow rate that most patients can accomplish. Normal values of the fraction of exhaled NO (FeNO) vary widely in both healthy and diseased populations depending on, for example, age, sex and smoking status. Exhaled NO levels are therefore generally interpreted in terms of cut points in patients with symptoms that suggest airway inflammation (Table 3.4).

High levels of exhaled NO indicate eosinophilic inflammation, which is likely to respond to corticosteroid therapy. Therefore, in patients with asthma symptoms, a high level of exhaled NO would suggest the need for additional corticosteroid therapy or to check adherence to current regimens. By contrast, low levels of exhaled NO indicate poorer corticosteroid responsiveness, and in some patients it may be appropriate to consider a dose reduction. Interpretation of indeterminate levels of

TABLE 3.4

**Cut points for the range of exhaled nitric oxide measurements and their interpretation**

|  | Adults (ppb) | Children (ppb) | Interpretation |
|---|---|---|---|
| Low | < 25 | < 20 | Eosinophilic inflammation less likely |
| Indeterminate | > 25 – < 50 | > 20 – < 35 | Indeterminate: interpret in clinical context |
| High | > 50 | > 35 | Eosinophilic inflammation likely |

NO, nitric oxide. ppb, parts per billion.
Adapted from Dweik RA et al. 2011.

exhaled NO depend on the clinical context and may be most useful for modulating the corticosteroid dose over time. In allergic asthma, high levels of exhaled NO may also suggest ongoing allergen exposure.

Exhaled NO levels are generally highly sensitive to corticosteroid treatments, but in corticosteroid-naive patients high levels of NO may be used to support a diagnosis of asthma, while low levels render an asthma diagnosis less likely.

## Allergen skin-prick tests and other tests for atopy

Skin-prick tests with allergens or detection of allergen-specific immunoglobulin (Ig)E in the circulation are the most common diagnostic tests for allergy. For the diagnosis of asthma, the results should always be interpreted in relation to the patient's history and the relationship between asthma symptoms and allergen exposure, because up to 45% of the population may exhibit atopy but only a proportion of these individuals will have asthma. Nevertheless, the identification of allergens that may be contributing to persistent asthma and exacerbations is important in order to provide advice on allergen avoidance or other treatment strategies. New molecular-level characterization of IgE specificity to a large number of allergens in a single test is an exciting new diagnostic development. However, a positive response to any single allergen must be interpreted in the clinical context and not in isolation.

## Patient groups

The diagnosis of asthma may be difficult in certain patient groups, especially smokers and the extremely young or old, who may have difficulty performing lung function tests. Individuals with other lung disease may also provide a mixed pattern on spirometry testing.

**Infants** may have recurrent wheezing due to acute viral respiratory infections; the first episode of wheezing in infants under the age of 6 months is usually due to viral bronchiolitis, whereas asthma is more likely to be the cause of wheezing after 18 months of age. After a viral infection, symptoms may persist in children with atopic asthma and a positive interaction between virus infection and sensitization to aeroallergens has been shown in genetically susceptible children.

Similarly, older children may show asthma symptoms in association with viral infections (exacerbation) or exercise; asthma should be considered if the child has a persistent nocturnal cough, or if colds go to the chest easily or take longer than 10 days to resolve.

**Asthma in older people.** In older people, asthma may coexist with conditions such as COPD, bronchiectasis, heart failure or interstitial pulmonary fibrosis. A history of asthma in childhood and variability on spirometry or PEF testing with $\beta_2$-agonists supports the diagnosis. However, late-onset asthma is often confused with COPD and an oral corticosteroid trial for up to 2 weeks with careful monitoring is a useful diagnostic discriminator.

**Occupational asthma** is also often misdiagnosed as chronic bronchitis or COPD. Ideally, diagnosis requires a detailed occupational history and the demonstration of a clear relationship between the development of symptoms at work and resolution of symptoms away from work.

**Seasonal asthma** associated with very high levels of aeroallergens may present as intermittent symptoms, with the patient being asymptomatic between seasons, or as seasonal worsening of moderate or severe asthma. Examples of seasonal asthma are the allergic rhinitis ('hay fever') and asthma that accompany the ragweed, parietaria, birch or cedar pollen seasons, in accordance with geographical location, experienced in well-defined periods of the calendar by pollen-sensitive individuals. Care must also be taken not to miss fungus-associated seasonal asthma (e.g. associated with *Alternaria* spp., *Cladasporium* spp. and *Aspergillus* spp.).

**Cough-variant asthma.** Patients present with cough as the principal symptom; they seldom wheeze. Coughing is often confined to the night, and examination during the day may not reveal evidence of abnormalities. Lung function tests and measurement of bronchial responsiveness with some form of challenge test are particularly important in these patients. Another helpful sign is eosinophils in the sputum but one form of this variant manifests with little airway reversibility or airway hyperresponsiveness (eosinophilic bronchitis).

## Differential diagnosis

Wheezing can arise from either widespread or localized airway obstruction, and this should be considered in the differential diagnosis (Figure 3.3). Breathlessness and cough are common symptoms of many conditions. The keys to diagnosing asthma are the patient's history together with measurements of lung function through spirometry and airway variability. An obstructive ventilatory defect alone suggests asthma or COPD while excluding other conditions. In adults, asthma-like symptoms can result from bronchitis or COPD; concomitant asthma and COPD are common among past or present smokers, and even occur in some individuals who have never smoked. Demonstration of reversible and variable airflow limitation confirms the diagnosis of asthma and indicates a trial of preventive treatment.

Although it is not always possible to distinguish asthma and COPD in those with a fixed component of airflow obstruction, detection of airflow obstruction warrants a trial of therapy with inhaled corticosteroids to assess reversibility and asthma still appears to be the most likely diagnosis in middle-aged adults (Figure 3.4).

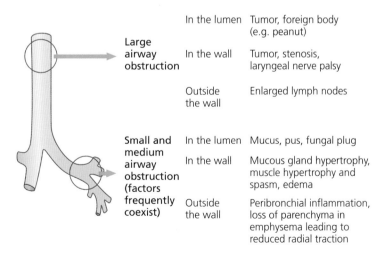

**Figure 3.3** Differential diagnosis of obstructive airway disease. Reproduced with permission from Professor Martyn R Partridge, Imperial College London.

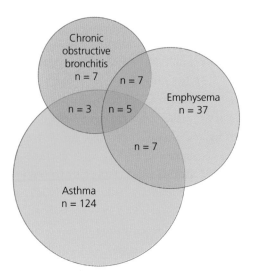

**Figure 3.4** The distribution of obstructive airways disease in a middle-aged population. While COPD and emphysema are present, reversible airflow obstruction (asthma) was the most common cause of airflow obstruction in this group of patients. Reproduced with permission from Abramson M. *MJA* 2005;183(1 suppl):S23–5.

## Classification of asthma severity

A combination of symptom measurements and lung function tests can be used to classify asthma according to its severity (Figure 3.5). These clinical measures of disease severity have been shown to correlate well with pathological markers of airway inflammation such as eosinophil numbers. However, classification of asthma by severity is not necessarily predictive of the amount or types of treatment required to achieve best asthma outcomes. Recent research using non-hierarchical and cluster approaches to diagnosis are identifying multiple disease phenotypes with varying inflammatory and cytokine profiles and differing physiological features, responses to treatment and natural histories. This level of complexity has yet to translate into treatment strategies, leaving us with treatment algorithms based on asthma control: an assessment of daytime and night-time symptoms, limitation of activities, the need for rescue reliever therapy, lung function, and exacerbation frequency and severity (see Chapter 4).

**Step 4: severe persistent**
- Symptoms daily
- Frequent exacerbations
- Frequent nocturnal asthma symptoms
- Limitation of physical activities
- $FEV_1$ or PEF ≤ 60% predicted
- PEF or $FEV_1$ variability > 30%

**Step 3: moderate persistent**
- Symptoms daily
- Exacerbations may affect activity and sleep
- Nocturnal symptoms more than once a week
- Daily use of inhaled short-acting $\beta_2$-agonist
- $FEV_1$ or PEF 60–80% predicted
- PEF or $FEV_1$ variability > 30%

**Step 2: mild persistent**
- Symptoms more than once a week but less than once a day
- Exacerbations may affect activity and sleep
- Nocturnal symptoms more than twice a month
- $FEV_1$ or PEF ≥ 80% predicted
- PEF or $FEV_1$ variability < 20–30%

**Step 1: intermittent**
- Symptoms less than once a week
- Brief exacerbations
- Nocturnal symptoms not more than twice a month
- $FEV_1$ or PEF ≥ 80% predicted
- PEF or $FEV_1$ variability < 20%

**Figure 3.5** Whilst classification of asthma severity is made in treated patients according to the treatment needed to control symptoms and exacerbations, in untreated patients severity may be classified as above. The worst feature determines the classification of severity. $FEV_1$, forced expiratory volume in 1 second; PEF, peak expiratory flow.

When assessing the severity of illness it is important to remember that patients often have a poor perception of the potential severity of their asthma, largely because they have adapted their lifestyle to accommodate their disease. There is also often a lack of lung function measurements to provide more objective information. It is important to recognize that even mild asthma can be associated with severe, potentially fatal exacerbations. Risk factors that have been shown to be associated with an increased risk of death from asthma include:

- a previous history of acute life-threatening attacks
- hospitalization for asthma within the previous year
- psychosocial problems
- a history of invasive ventilation for asthma
- recent reduction or cessation of systemic corticosteroid therapy
- non-adherence to preventive treatments
- difficulty accessing treatment.

Conversely, a written asthma action plan has been found to be protective against asthma death.

## Key points – diagnosis and classification

- Although asthma is one of the most common chronic disorders, it is often underdiagnosed or misdiagnosed.
- The clinical diagnosis of asthma is often based on the presence of symptoms, such as breathlessness (often episodic), wheezing, chest tightness and coughing.
- A key feature is variation of symptoms over time, especially diurnal variation.
- Objective measures of lung function are important in order to establish asthma as a diagnosis and to assess response to treatment.
- Measurement of bronchial responsiveness and allergy status can aid diagnosis as well as identify possible exacerbating factors.
- Attempts should be made to assess disease control to guide treatment.
- The diagnosis of asthma may be difficult in certain patient groups, particularly those who smoke and the very young or old.

## Key references

Chen H, Gould MK, Blanc PD et al. Asthma control, severity and quality of life: quantifying the effect of uncontrolled disease. *J Allergy Clin Immunol* 2007;120:396–402.

Dweik RA, Boggs PB, Erzurum SC et al. An official ATS clinical practice guideline: interpretation of exhaled nitric oxide levels (FeNO) for clinical applications. *Am J Respir Crit Care Med* 2011;184:602-15. Available at http://ajrccm.atsjournals.org/content/184/5/602.full.pdf.html, last accessed 14 February 2013.

Global Initiative for Asthma. *Global Strategy for Asthma Management and Prevention; Updated 2012.* Available from www.ginasthma.org, last accessed 12 March 2013.

Green RH, Brightling CE, McKenna S et al. Asthma exacerbations and sputum eosinophil counts: a randomised controlled trial. *Lancet* 2002;360:1715–21.

Haldar P, Pavord ID. Noneosinophilic asthma: a distinct clinical and pathologic phenotype. *J Allergy Clin Immunol* 2007;119:1043–52.

Johns DP, Pierce R. *Spirometry: The Measurement and Interpretation of Ventilatory Function in Clinical Practice*, 2008. www.nationalasthma.org.au/uploads/content/211-spirometer_handbook_naca.pdf, last accessed 02 January 2013.

Smith AD, Cowan JO, Brassett KP et al. Use of exhaled nitric oxide measurements to guide treatment in chronic asthma. *N Engl J Med* 2005;352:2163–73.

Successful asthma management will achieve both control of symptoms and prevention of acute attacks (Table 4.1). To achieve this, preventive measures including the use of medication to prevent symptoms to treat acute attacks is necessary. Avoidance of triggers where possible can also be important (see allergen avoidance in Chapter 6). Drugs used in the management of asthma can be classified as controllers (also called preventers) and relievers.

## Controller (preventer) medications

Controllers (preventers) are taken daily over the long term to control persistent asthma (Table 4.2). They include anti-inflammatory agents such as corticosteroids, sodium cromoglicate, nedocromil sodium and leukotriene modifiers, and long-acting bronchodilators such as long-acting $\beta_2$-agonists (LABAs), omalizumab and sustained-release theophylline.

**Inhaled corticosteroids,** such as beclometasone (beclomethasone) dipropionate, budesonide, fluticasone propionate, mometasone, fluticasone furoate and ciclesonide, are the most effective anti-inflammatory agents currently available for asthma management. They are the mainstay of effective asthma treatment, improving symptoms

---

TABLE 4.1

**Aims of asthma management**

- Control symptoms
- Prevent exacerbations
- Maintain pulmonary function as close to normal levels as possible
- Maintain normal levels of activity
- Prevent the development of irreversible airflow limitation
- Prevent asthma mortality

TABLE 4.2

**Effects of anti-asthma drugs and risks of serious adverse events during long-term use**

| | Control of symptoms over weeks to months | Relief of exacerbations over minutes or hours | Risk of serious long-term adverse events |
|---|---|---|---|
| Inhaled corticosteroids | +++ | − | + (at high doses) |
| Oral corticosteroids (prednisolone) | ++ | ++ (over hours) | +++ |
| Sodium cromoglicate | + | − | − |
| Nedocromil sodium | + | − | − |
| Leukotriene modifiers | ++ | + | − |
| Short-acting inhaled $\beta_2$-agonists | +/− | +++ | − |
| Long-acting inhaled $\beta_2$-agonists | ++ | ++/+++ | − |
| Oral $\beta_2$-agonists | +/− | + | + |
| Theophylline | | + | ++ |
| Omalizumab | | ++ | − |
| Inhaled anticholinergic agents | + | ++ | − |

and preventing exacerbations, and their use is associated with protection from asthma deaths. Studies have consistently shown that these agents reduce pathological signs of airway inflammation, so that lung function and symptoms improve, bronchial hyperresponsiveness decreases, and the frequency and severity of exacerbations are reduced. Corticosteroids interrupt the signaling pathways for pro-inflammatory molecules by decreasing the expression of genes for a variety of inflammatory mediators and by increasing the expression of genes for anti-inflammatory mediators.

Inhaled corticosteroids are also useful in the treatment of persistent asthma because they reduce the need for oral corticosteroids and have fewer systemic adverse effects. Local adverse effects, which include oropharyngeal candidiasis, dysphonia and coughing, can largely be prevented by using spacer devices and mouth rinsing after use. Potential systemic adverse effects include thinning of the skin, cataract formation, adrenal suppression and decreased bone metabolism and growth. The risk of such effects depends on a number of factors, including the dose taken, absorption from the gut or lung, the extent of first-pass metabolism in the gut wall and liver, and the half-life of the corticosteroid. In general, the risk of significant systemic effects is low with therapeutic doses.

The recommended doses of inhaled corticosteroids depend on the type of medication and inhaler used. By convention, inhaled corticosteroid doses are presented as equivalent doses of beclometasone dipropionate. It is also evident that the majority of benefits of inhaled corticosteroids are achieved at low to medium doses, with the risks of inhaled corticosteroid medication increasing at higher doses.

**Systemic corticosteroids**, such as prednisolone, can be given either orally or parenterally. Short courses (3–7 days) can be used when starting therapy in patients with uncontrolled asthma or during periods of worsening asthma. Long-term treatment may rarely be necessary in patients with severe persistent asthma; patients who require such medication should be seen by a specialist. Systemic events associated with oral corticosteroids include impairment of growth in children, osteoporosis, arterial hypertension, adrenal suppression, obesity, thinning of the skin, muscle weakness, cataract formation and diabetes. It should be noted that long-term inhaled corticosteroid therapy is far safer than oral or parenteral corticosteroid therapy.

**Leukotriene modifiers.** The cysteinyl leukotrienes (cysLTs) – $LTC_4$, $LTD_4$, and $LTE_4$, – are potent mediators of asthma. They are generated from arachidonic acid by the 5-lipoxygenase pathway that operates in mast cells and eosinophils. Once known as 'slow-reacting substance of anaphylaxis', cysLTs released during the inflammatory process cause prolonged contraction of smooth muscle, microvascular leakage, mucus secretion and eosinophil attraction. As the structure of the leukotrienes was elucidated in 1979, a number of leukotriene-modifying drugs have been developed and introduced into the market. Zafirlukast, montelukast and pranlukast are anti-asthma drugs that inhibit the effect of leukotrienes at their receptor (cysteinyl leukotriene receptor, cysLTR1). In addition, inhibitors of 5-lipoxygenase, such as zileuton, interrupt the conversion of arachidonic acid into leukotrienes, including the cysLTs and LTB4.

Treatment with one of these oral drugs can produce improvement in pulmonary function, protection from exercise-induced asthma and reduced eosinophilic inflammation. A clinical response is usually seen within 3 weeks of therapy, though not all patients benefit. Patients with asthma associated with intolerance to acetylsalicylic acid (ASA; aspirin) and other non-steroidal anti-inflammatory drugs (NSAIDs) seem to be particularly responsive.

Leukotriene modifiers can be used to treat mild persistent asthma, especially in children for whom the use of inhaled corticosteroids is limited because of concerns regarding the effects on growth. However, these drugs are less effective overall than a low dose of inhaled corticosteroid. They can also be used together with an inhaled corticosteroid in moderate and severe asthma, but are less effective than the combination of an inhaled corticosteroid and an inhaled LABA. Clearly, the advantages of these drugs over other long-term controllers (preventers) are that they are orally administered and are not corticosteroids; patient acceptability and adherence is therefore likely to be good.

**Sodium cromoglicate and nedocromil sodium.** Inhaled sodium cromoglicate and nedocromil sodium inhibit allergen-induced airflow limitation and acute airflow limitation after exercise or exposure to cold air or sulfur dioxide. They work by stabilizing mast cells and sensory nerves by stimulating the newly identified GP receptor 35. Each agent can be used as long-term therapy early in the course of asthma; a course of 4–6 weeks may be needed to determine effectiveness in a given patient. Adverse effects are few, though coughing may result from inhalation of the powder formulation. Both agents can be used as maintenance therapy for asthma but are less effective than a low dose of inhaled corticosteroids. As these agents have few side effects, they have found particular use in childhood asthma.

**Sustained-release theophylline.** Theophylline is a bronchodilator, and there is some evidence that it may also have anti-inflammatory effects. It is both an inhibitor of cyclic adenosine 5'-monophosphate (cAMP) phosphodiesterase and an antagonist of adenosine purinoreceptors. During long-term treatment, sustained-release theophylline controls symptoms and improves lung function. Because of its long duration of action, it is useful in controlling nocturnal symptoms that persist despite regular anti-inflammatory treatment. However, theophylline has a number of potentially serious adverse effects (Table 4.3); theophylline intoxication can result in seizures and death. Furthermore, the drug has a relatively narrow therapeutic index; serum concentrations producing adverse effects are close to those required for therapeutic efficacy. Appropriate dosing and monitoring are therefore essential; in general, dosing should produce a steady-state serum theophylline concentration of 5–15 µg/mL. Monitoring is advisable when treatment is started and at regular intervals thereafter. In addition, serum drug concentrations should be monitored if:

- adverse events occur with the usual dose
- the expected therapeutic benefit is not achieved

TABLE 4.3

**Adverse effects associated with theophylline**

| | |
|---|---|
| • Nausea | • Arrhythmias |
| • Vomiting | • Headache |
| • Gastrointestinal disturbances | • Insomnia |
| • Tachycardia | • Convulsions |
| • Palpitations | |

- the patient has a condition that is likely to affect theophylline metabolism (e.g. febrile illness, pregnancy, liver disease, congestive heart failure)
- the patient is receiving concomitant treatment with drugs that interact with theophylline (e.g. cimetidine, some quinolone antibiotics).

**Long-acting $\beta_2$-agonists** such as salmeterol xinafoate and formoterol fumarate dihydrate, have a duration of action of more than 12 hours. They act by relaxing airway smooth muscle, enhancing mucociliary clearance and decreasing vascular permeability; in addition, they may modulate mediator release from mast cells and basophils. Long-term treatment with inhaled preparations of LABAs improves symptoms and lung function, relieves nocturnal asthma and reduces the need for short-acting $\beta_2$-agonists (SABAs). Such preparations can be used as a more effective alternative to increasing the corticosteroid dose in patients for whom standard starting doses of inhaled corticosteroids do not control symptoms. A LABA should not be given without an inhaled corticosteroid for asthma as studies have suggested this to be associated with an increase in mortality. Combination therapies of inhaled corticosteroids and LABAs are now widely used (see page 60). Adverse events associated with LABAs include cardiovascular stimulation, anxiety, heartburn and tremor.

**Omalizumab** is a humanized monoclonal IgG anti-IgE antibody, which is administered every 2–4 weeks by subcutaneous injection. The dose is titrated according to body weight and the serum level of total IgE. It binds to the part of the IgE molecule that attaches to the high-affinity and low-affinity receptors on mediator-secreting cells, thereby depriving the cells of the necessary allergen-specific IgE required to trigger secretion of mediators. The net result is that the serum level of free IgE drops steeply with the first injection and then gradually, over several weeks, IgE in the airways also falls, followed by downregulation of IgE receptors. Generally, an effect is observed after 4–6 months of treatment with attenuation of both early- and late-phase allergen-induced bronchoconstriction in parallel with a reduction in airway inflammation, including a decrease in airway eosinophils.

Clinical trials have revealed that this anti-allergy treatment is effective in treating allergic asthma. The availability of omalizumab is limited by its expense, but the drug is considered cost-effective in the management of severe and chronic asthma, particularly in reducing exacerbations and hospitalizations. Currently, omalizumab is listed as appropriate for Step 5 asthma treatment (from GINA guidelines, see Figure 4.6): that is, for patients who have poorly controlled asthma despite maximal doses of inhaled corticosteroids and LABAs. In order to avoid non-responsive patients receiving omalizumab, a 16-week trial of therapy is recommended, after which the clinician is asked to assess responsiveness using multiple endpoints. The major side effect of this drug has been the uncommon occurrence of anaphylaxis and severe asthma episodes following administration, which can occur several hours after the injection. Consequently, most treatment guidelines recommend observing the patient for 1–2 hours after administration and provision of an anaphylaxis plan and an epinephrine (adrenaline) auto-injector for patients to take home with them.

## Reliever medications

Relievers (sometimes referred to as rescue medication) are used to rapidly reverse the bronchoconstriction and associated symptoms during acute attacks (see Table 4.2). They include SABAs, LABAs with a rapid onset of action, short-acting theophylline and short-acting anticholinergic agents. The most effective forms are those that are delivered by inhalation directly to the airways.

**Short-acting $\beta_2$-agonists.** Inhaled SABAs, such as salbutamol and terbutaline, are used to control bronchoconstriction, and are the treatment of choice for the management of acute exacerbations and the prophylaxis of exercise-induced asthma. Oral preparations are also available and may be suitable for patients who are unable to use inhaled medication. In general, oral administration is less desirable than inhaled administration because systemic side effects such as tachycardia are more pronounced when the drug is delivered orally.

Concern has been expressed over the long-term safety of repeatedly inhaling short-acting $\beta_2$-bronchodilators. Several points are worth making in relation to the use of these quick relievers. They are certainly the best drugs for relieving acute bronchospasm and associated symptoms, but their increased use by a patient is a sign of worsening asthma and the need for greater use of controller (preventer) drugs. The use of one canister of a metered-dose inhaler per month should certainly sound alarm bells. Regular use of SABAs is not recommended, as a refractory response may develop, and it has been suggested that asthma may worsen. In addition, it is now known that genetic $\beta_2$-adrenoceptor polymorphisms influence the effectiveness of these drugs, particularly with regard to tachyphylaxis or the development of refractoriness; therefore SABAs should only be used for quick relief on an 'as-required' basis.

**Long-acting $\beta_2$-agonists** with a rapid onset of action (e.g. formoterol) can be used as bronchodilators to treat acute asthma symptoms. Because of the concerns regarding the use of a LABA without an inhaled corticosteroid, this form of therapy is usually provided in an inhaler combined with an inhaled corticosteroid.

**Systemic corticosteroids.** Oral corticosteroid preparations have a relatively slow onset of action (4–6 hours), but are extremely useful in the treatment of severe acute exacerbations because they prevent progression of the exacerbation. As a result, they also reduce the need for emergency treatment or hospitalization, prevent early relapse and reduce the morbidity associated with exacerbations. Treatment is normally continued for 3–10 days after the exacerbation; the dose can be reduced and stopped as symptoms resolve and lung function returns to the personal best level.

**Anticholinergic agents.** Inhaled anticholinergic agents such as ipratropium bromide or oxitropium bromide cause bronchodilatation by inhibiting postganglionic efferent vagal fibers, thereby reducing the vagal tone of the airways. They also inhibit reflex bronchoconstriction provoked by inhaled irritants. They are less effective than inhaled $\beta_2$-agonists and have a slower onset of action, taking 30–60 minutes to reach their maximum effect. They are particularly useful when administered as a nebulized aqueous aerosol in acute severe asthma exacerbations and as long-term therapy for patients with chronic obstructive pulmonary disease (COPD). Adverse effects include dry mouth and a bad taste.

**Short-acting theophylline.** Oral treatment with short-acting theophylline has been used for pretreatment of exercise-induced asthma and for symptomatic relief. The role of theophylline in the treatment of exacerbations is controversial and, because of the high risk of adverse effects and the slow onset of action, it is now rarely used in developed countries except for acute severe life-threatening asthma.

**Combination therapy.** A series of clinical trials have shown that the inhaled LABAs salmeterol and formoterol, when administered to patients who are already taking inhaled corticosteroids but whose asthma is poorly controlled, may produce greater improvements in pulmonary function and symptom control than would be obtained by doubling the dose of inhaled corticosteroid. Combinations of an inhaled corticosteroid and a LABA – specifically, fluticasone propionate and salmeterol, budesonide and formoterol and fluticasone propionate and formoterol – are now available in single inhalers. The addition of a LABA is indicated for all whose asthma fails to be controlled with low-dose inhaled corticosteroid. It would seem, therefore, that the dose–response curve for topical corticosteroids is not linear, and that the overall benefits obtained with doses of up to approximately 400 µg HFA-beclometasone dipropionate per day or equivalent are as great as those that can be achieved with further increments (HFA refers to the propellant hydrofluoroalkane-134a). One possible explanation for these observations is that topical corticosteroids are able to control the inflammatory response by inhibiting cytokine and other relevant pathways. They are not able to alter, at least in the short and medium term, the behavior of the remodeled airway with its increased smooth muscle, microvasculature and thickened airway walls. In this situation, drugs that act on the airway smooth muscle and microvasculature to restore airway physiology to normal, such as a LABA, are likely to be effective.

All controller and reliever combination medications are indicated to be taken regularly, usually twice daily, as a preventative for asthma exacerbation and to control the underlying airway inflammation characteristic of asthma.

The formulation of budesonide and formoterol combination treatment can be used as a single inhaler to deliver both maintenance preventive treatment as well as being used as a reliever. This means patients have only one inhaler for both their controller and reliever therapy. Some trials indicate that this approach can be effective in preventing exacerbations as patients will receive increased inhaled corticosteroid as well as bronchodilator therapy at the first sign of worsening symptoms as they use their reliever medications. Currently, the only single inhaler approach to demonstrate effective regular preventer and as-needed reliever therapy in clinical studies is the budesonide/formoterol combination inhaler as formoterol (unlike salmeterol) has a rapid onset of action, enabling its use as a reliever medication in a single-inhaler treatment plan.

## Delivery of inhaled medication

Inhalation of aerosols or powders achieves high drug concentrations in the airways and reduces the risk of systemic adverse effects. A variety of delivery devices are available (Table 4.4). Whichever device is chosen, its use should be explained carefully to the patient (Figures 4.1 and 4.2), and the patient's technique checked regularly.

**Pressurized metered-dose inhalers** (pMDIs) are the most widely used type of inhaler, delivering a measured dose of medication. Delivery is efficient when the device is used correctly (see Figure 4.1).

Many patients, however, are unable to coordinate inspiration with inhaler actuation. The use of a spacer device (Figures 4.3–4.5) can overcome this problem and also reduces oropharyngeal deposition of

61

TABLE 4.4

**Devices for delivery of aerosolized medication in asthma**

- Pressurized metered-dose inhalers (pMDIs)
- Breath-actuated pMDIs (e.g. Autohaler)
- Dry-powder inhalers (e.g. Accuhaler, Diskhaler, Easyhaler, Rotahaler, Spinhaler, Turbohaler*)
- Spacer devices (e.g. AeroChamber, Babyhaler, Nebuhaler, Volumatic)
- Nebulizers

*Turbuhaler in some countries.

drug and the incidence of local side effects. The use of a spacer for delivery of all medication through a pMDI, especially controller therapy, is recommended. The medication is discharged into the spacer and held in suspension for several seconds. During this time, the patient can inhale the drug in one or several breaths, without the need to coordinate inspiration and drug delivery; this may be particularly useful in small children and patients with poor coordination. A small-volume spacer can be adapted with a face mask for young children. The use of spacers also allows high doses to be given during attacks, eight to 12 puffs of reliever medication in a pMDI being indicated

Some pMDIs are constituted to release very fine particles on activation of the inhaler, and thus achieve improved drug deposition and efficacy, especially to the periphery of the lung. This increases systemic bioavailability from lung absorption and consequently increases the risk of side effects unless the dose is adjusted accordingly.

**Breath-actuated inhalers,** in which the valve is actuated during inspiration, are useful in patients who have difficulty coordinating actuation and breathing. Drug deposition appears to be greater than with pMDIs.

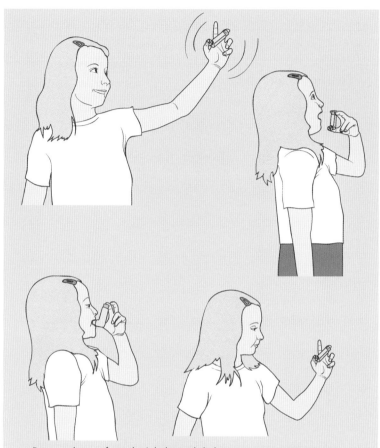

- Remove the cap from the inhaler and shake
- Breathe out gently
- Put the mouthpiece between the teeth and close lips around the mouthpiece to form a good seal
- Start to breathe in slowly through the mouth and press to actuate the puffer; continue to breathe in slowly and deeply
- Hold breath for up to 10 seconds or for as long as is comfortable
- While holding breath, remove the inhaler from mouth
- Breathe out gently
- If an extra dose is needed, wait 1 minute before repeating; replace cap

**Figure 4.1** Technique for use of a metered-dose inhaler without a spacer device.

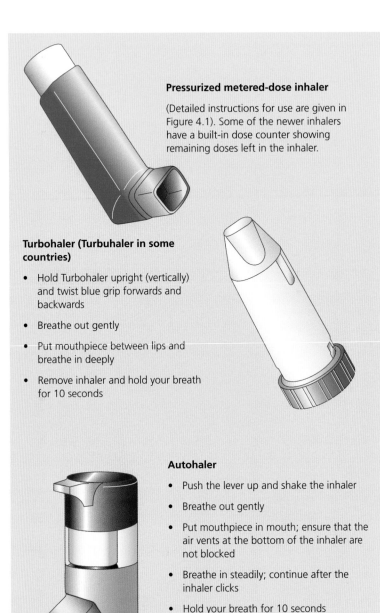

**Pressurized metered-dose inhaler**

(Detailed instructions for use are given in Figure 4.1). Some of the newer inhalers have a built-in dose counter showing remaining doses left in the inhaler.

**Turbohaler (Turbuhaler in some countries)**

- Hold Turbohaler upright (vertically) and twist blue grip forwards and backwards
- Breathe out gently
- Put mouthpiece between lips and breathe in deeply
- Remove inhaler and hold your breath for 10 seconds

**Autohaler**

- Push the lever up and shake the inhaler
- Breathe out gently
- Put mouthpiece in mouth; ensure that the air vents at the bottom of the inhaler are not blocked
- Breathe in steadily; continue after the inhaler clicks
- Hold your breath for 10 seconds
- Lower lever on inhaler
- Wait at least 60 seconds before taking the next inhalation

**Figure 4.2** Different inhaler devices and instructions for their use.

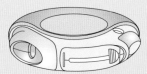

### Accuhaler (Diskus)

- Hold the outer casing in one hand while pushing the thumb grip away until you hear a click

- With the mouthpiece towards you, slide the lever away until it clicks; this makes the dose available and moves the counter on

- Breathe out gently away from the mouthpiece, then put mouthpiece in mouth and breathe in

- Remove inhaler and hold your breath for 10 seconds

- Close by sliding thumb grip back towards you until it clicks

### Diskhaler

To load:

- Remove mouthpiece cover; pull the tray out gently until you can squeeze the ridges on each side and slide it out

- Place the foil disk on the wheel, numbers upwards, and slide the tray back

- Hold the corners of the tray and slide it in and out to rotate the disk until the highest number (8 or 4) shows in the window

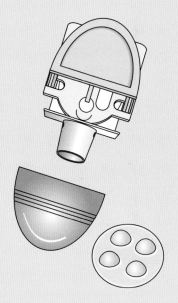

To use:

- Keeping the Diskhaler level, raise the rear of the lid as far as it will go so that the pin pierces the blister in the disk

- Still keeping the Diskhaler level, breathe out gently, put mouthpiece in mouth and breathe in as deeply as possible; do not block the two small air vents on the sides of the mouthpiece

- Remove Diskhaler from mouth and hold your breath for 10 seconds

- Slide tray in and out to prepare next dose

**Figure 4.2** *continued*

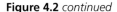

**Easyhaler**

- Open the protective cover
- Remove the dust cap from the Easyhaler mouthpiece
- Shake the Easyhaler vigorously
- Hold in the upright position and push down the actuator until it clicks
- Keeping the Easyhaler upright let the actuator click back up
- Breathe out fully; place the Easyhaler mouthpiece between teeth and seal lips tightly around it
- Take a full, deep breath in, and hold your breath for at least 5 seconds
- Remove the Easyhaler from mouth, shake and repeat actuation steps above for a second dose if needed
- Replace the dust cap and protective cover

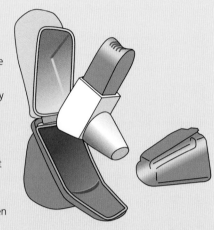

Note: the dose counter will go red when you have 20 doses left. Clean the mouthpiece weekly with a clean cloth or tissue. If using the Easyhaler for controller treatments rinse your mouth after taking your medication.

**Figure 4.2** *continued*

(a)                                  (b)

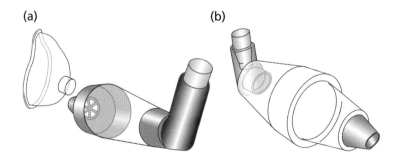

**Figure 4.3** Spacer devices for use by (a) young children who need assistance and (b) patients who can use the device without help.

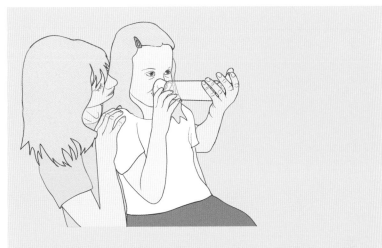

- Shake the inhaler and insert it into the spacer
- Put the mouthpiece into the child's mouth and seal the child's lips around the mouthpiece
- The child should breathe in and out slowly and gently
- Depress the canister as the child breathes in and out: one puff for at least every four breath cycles
- Remove the spacer from the child's mouth
- Generally, two puffs is adequate – this can be repeated every few minutes in acute severe asthma (see Chapter 5)

**Figure 4.4** Use of a spacer by a young child – instructions for parents/carers.

**Dry-powder inhalers** (DPIs) require a different inhalation technique from that needed with pMDIs. No propellant is needed because the drug is released by inspiratory airflow. However, a certain minimum flow rate is required, and thus these devices may be less effective in young children, during severe attacks and in those with very poor lung function. Inhalation of dry particles can cause coughing.

**Nebulizers** generate a wet aerosol by blowing compressed air through a drug solution or suspension, or by ultrasonic vibration. The patient inhales the aerosol through a face mask or mouthpiece. Nebulizers have largely been replaced in emergency settings and for young children by pMDIs and spacers, which have demonstrated equivalent

67

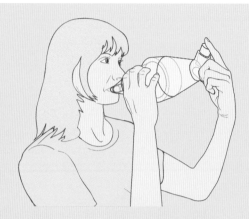

- Shake inhaler and insert it into the spacer
- Put the mouthpiece in your mouth
- Press the canister and breathe in slowly and deeply
- Hold your breath for 10 seconds*
- Breathe out through the mouthpiece
- Breathe in again, but do not press the canister this time
- Remove the device and wait for 30 seconds before taking another inhalation

*Alternatively, breathe normally through the spacer for at least four breaths.

**Figure 4.5** Use of a spacer by a patient who can operate it without help.

drug delivery. This removes the need to purchase a nebulizer and air pump, and avoids the problems of portability of this equipment in an emergency or to remote settings. Nebulized therapy is still used for those with very severe lung disease or extreme attacks. A standard dose of nebulized $\beta_2$-agonist is equivalent to eight to 12 puffs from a pMDI and spacer.

## Asthma control

There are two broad aims of asthma control. The first is to reduce or eliminate asthma symptoms or the limitations of activities due to asthma. Key elements in assessing asthma control include the presence of symptoms both by day and night, the requirement for reliever medication and lung function or peak flow measurements. While assessment of symptoms can occur in the process of a clinical consultation, questionnaires have been developed to reliably measure asthma control, such as the Asthma Control Questionnaire (ACQ) or the Asthma Control Test (ACT). These can be used by both clinicians and patients to gain a reliable and longitudinal record of control of symptoms (Table 4.5)

The second aim of asthma control is prevention of exacerbations. While achieving control of asthma symptoms is likely to lead to prevention of exacerbations in most, for some patients asthma exacerbations are the predominant feature of their asthma. As asthma exacerbations can be life-threatening and are inevitably disruptive to patients and their carers, in these instances prevention of exacerbations should be the major focus of treatment. Factors indicating a high risk for future exacerbations include a past history of severe or life-threatening asthma attack, exacerbation occurring despite adequate preventative treatment, impaired interval lung function and cigarette smoke exposure.

## Stepwise approach to asthma treatment

Current management guidelines recommend a stepwise approach to asthma treatment, depending on disease control (Table 4.5), in both adults and children (Figure 4.6). All patients should aim to have well-controlled asthma, and treatment should be stepped up or down, as appropriate, every 1–3 months to achieve and maintain asthma control.

Recommended management strategies suggest five treatment steps. Patients should be started on therapy appropriate to the initial level of symptoms: step 2 is appropriate for most patients who are receiving no, or only as-needed, bronchodilator treatment for asthma, and step 3 is appropriate for those with more uncontrolled symptoms and reduced lung function at the start of treatment.

Depending on symptom severity and the presence of exacerbations, treatment should be continued at a given level for 1–3 months before considering escalation or reduction. Generally, after 3 months of well-controlled asthma a step down to a lower level of treatment should be considered.

TABLE 4.5

**Levels of asthma control**

A: Assessment of current clinical control (preferably over 4 weeks)

| Symptom | Controlled (all of the following) | Partly controlled (any measure present) | Uncontrolled |
|---|---|---|---|
| Daytime symptoms | None (twice or less/week) | More than twice/week | Three or more features of partly controlled asthma*[†] |
| Limitation of activities | None | Any | |
| Nocturnal symptoms/ awakening | None | Any | |
| Need for reliever/ rescue reliever treatment | None (twice or less/week) | More than twice/ week | |
| Lung function (PEF or FEV$_1$)[‡] | Normal | < 80% predicted or personal best (if known) | |

B : Assessment of future risk (risk of exacerbations, instability, rapid decline in lung function, side effects)

Features that are associated with increased risk of adverse events in the future include:

- poor clinical control
- frequent exacerbations in past year
- ever admission to a critical care unit for asthma
- low FEV$_1$
- exposure to cigarette smoke
- high-dose medications

*Any exacerbation should prompt review of maintenance treatment to ensure that it is adequate.
[†]By definition, an exacerbation in any week makes that an uncontrolled asthma week.
[‡]Without administration of bronchodilator, lung function is not a reliable test for children 5 years and younger.
Reproduced with permission from Global Initiative for Asthma, 2012.

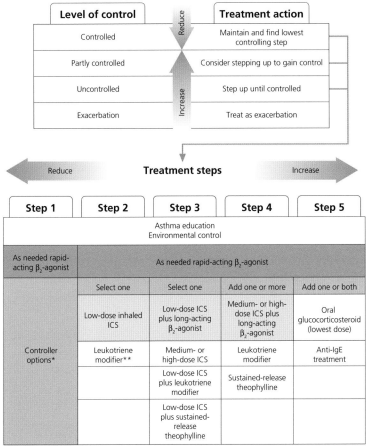

*Preferred controller options are shown in shaded boxes
**Receptor antagonist or synthesis inhibitors

Alternative reliever treatments include inhaled anticholinergics, short-acting oral $\beta_2$-agonists, some long-acting $\beta_2$-agonists, and short-acting theophylline. Regular dosing with short- and long-acting $\beta_2$-agonist is not advised unless accompanied by regular use of an inhaled glucocorticosteroid.

**Figure 4.6** Stepwise approach to the long-term management of asthma in children older than 5 years, adolescents and adults. Patients should start treatment at steps 2 or 3 depending on their levels of symptoms and indicators of asthma severity. A rescue course of prednisolone may be needed at any time and any step. ICS, inhaled glucocorticosteroids; Ig, immunoglobulin. See Table 4.6 for ICS dose definitions. Reproduced with permission from the Global Initiative for Asthma, 2012.

**Step 1** is indicated for asthma with infrequent symptoms (less than twice a week) and normal interval lung function. For these patients, an inhaled as-needed SABA may be appropriate therapy without a regular controller treatment. Such patients can still experience exacerbations and the intensity of treatment for exacerbations should depend on the severity of the exacerbation (see Chapter 5).

**Step 2** is usually indicated for initial treatment in those who have moderate symptoms. It involves the regular use of a low-dose inhaled corticosteroid medication (Table 4.6) in addition to a rapidly acting $\beta_2$-agonist for symptom relief as needed. The dose of inhaled corticosteroid at this level would range from 200 to 500 µg daily of beclometasone or equivalent medication in adults, and 100 to 200 µg daily in children. While the best available evidence supports inhaled corticosteroids for asthma treatment at this level for prevention of exacerbations and symptom control, leukotriene modifiers are an alternative at this treatment step. Leukotriene modifier medication is particularly favored in children for whom the dose of inhaled corticosteroid needs to be minimized, although existing evidence suggests that leukotriene modifier medication is less effective in preventing exacerbations than low-dose inhaled corticosteroid medication.

TABLE 4.6

**Daily doses of inhaled corticosteroids: definitions for low, medium and high doses**

| Dose level | Beclometa- sone-HFA* | Fluticasone propionate* | Ciclesonide[†] | Budesonide* |
|---|---|---|---|---|
| Low | 100-200 µg | 100-200 µg | 80-160 µg | 200-400 µg |
| Medium | 200-400 µg | 200-400 µg | 160-320 µg | 400-800 µg |
| High | > 400 µg | > 400 µg | > 320 µg | > 800 µg |

*ex-valve dose. [†]ex-acuator dose. HFA-beclometasone is equivalent to twice the dose of CFC-containing beclometasone products.

Adapted from *Asthma Management Handbook 2006*. Melbourne: National Asthma Council Australia, 2006.

**Step 3.** Patients who still have symptoms of uncontrolled asthma despite using a low-dose inhaled corticosteroid, or those with more severe symptoms without treatment, should progress to step 3. This involves the addition of a LABA to regularly administered low-dose inhaled corticosteroid therapy and as-needed short-acting reliever therapy. The available evidence suggests that use of a LABA at this level provides symptom control superior to that from increasing doses of inhaled corticosteroids.

An alternative method of delivering therapy at this or later stages of management is a combined inhaled corticosteroid/LABA for both preventer and reliever therapy. This relies on the use of a rapid- and long-acting $\beta_2$-agonist (formoterol) in combination with a low-dose formulation of inhaled corticosteroid (usually budesonide, 200–400 µg twice daily) to be used as both controller and reliever therapy. This treatment has the advantage of convenience, as well as enabling the delivery of increased doses of inhaled corticosteroid for symptoms, thereby increasing anti-inflammatory controller treatment at the first sign of worsening symptoms. Evidence supports this approach for reducing asthma exacerbations. A potential concern with this approach is that patients may not take regular controller medication, and education therefore needs to emphasize the importance of using the budesonide/formoterol inhaler for both regular maintenance as well as reliever treatment.

At this treatment step, other options are the addition of a theophylline to low-dose inhaled corticosteroid medication or the addition of a leukotriene modifier, but both these treatment strategies appear to be less effective than the combination of a LABA with low-dose inhaled corticosteroid.

**Step 4.** Patients with more severe asthma and persistent symptoms despite step 3 treatment should be treated with escalating doses of inhaled corticosteroid and LABA therapy in addition to a SABA. Moderate to high doses of inhaled corticosteroid treatment are up to 1000 µg daily of HFA-beclometasone or equivalent in adults and up to 400 µg in children. At this level of treatment, additional controllers such as sustained-release theophylline or leukotriene modifiers can also be used.

> **Key points – management**
>
> • Drugs used in the management of asthma can be classified as controllers (preventers) or relievers: controllers are taken daily on a long-term basis to control persistent asthma; relievers are used to rapidly reverse the bronchoconstriction and associated symptoms during acute attacks.
> • Controllers (e.g. inhaled corticosteroids) are the mainstay of asthma therapy. Increased use of relievers (short-acting $\beta_2$-agonists) indicates inadequate disease control.
> • Asthma therapy should be tailored to disease severity; current management guidelines recommend a stepwise approach to treatment.
> • Any exacerbation should prompt a review of maintenance medications.
> • All patients with asthma should have a written asthma action plan.
> • If recommended treatment fails, adherence and diagnosis should be re-examined before treatment is escalated.

**Step 5.** The highest level of treatment, step 5, involves the addition of oral corticosteroid treatment and/or anti-IgE therapy for patients with uncontrolled asthma despite the use of high-dose controller inhaled corticosteroids and LABAs. Such unresponsive asthma symptoms should prompt a consideration of the diagnosis of asthma and the exclusion of other factors that may be worsening asthma. It is also appropriate to seek specialist referral at this stage. Oral corticosteroids should be used at the lowest dose and for the minimum time required to gain asthma symptom control. Immunosuppressants such as methotrexate, cyclophosphamide, ciclosporin, tacrolimus and azathioprine are occasionally used as oral corticosteroid-sparing agents.

**Infants and young children.** The symptom-driven stepwise approach to asthma care described above is similar in children. Generally, in very young children, low-dose inhaled corticosteroid treatments are preferred at step 2 of care. The dose ranges of inhaled corticosteroids should be considerably lower for children than for adults. Children over 7 years of age can usually use a puffer and spacer device, while those under 4 years of age are likely to require a face mask and spacer to deliver asthma treatments effectively. Between these ages the choice of device depends on the child and their experience with the medication.

**Written treatment plan.** All patients with asthma should have a written plan that describes their current step of asthma treatment and advises on treatment adjustments to accommodate worsening asthma (see Chapter 6). For many patients, such a plan will also involve instructions to take oral corticosteroids or seek medical advice for prescription of oral corticosteroid treatment.

### Key references

The Childhood Asthma Management Program Research Group. Long-term effects of budesonide or nedocromil in children with asthma. *N Engl J Med* 2000;343:1054–63.

Clark TJH, Godfrey S, Lee TH, eds. Asthma. 4th edn. London: Hodder Arnold, 2000.

Gibson PG, Powell H, Wilson A et al. Self-management education and regular practitioner review for adults with asthma (update). *Cochrane Database Syst Rev* 2003;(1):CD001117.

Global Initiative for Asthma. *Global Strategy for Asthma Management and Prevention; Updated 2012.* Available from www.ginasthma.org, last accessed 12 March 2013.

National Heart, Lung and Blood Institute. *Expert Panel Report 3: Guidelines for the Diagnosis and Management of Asthma.* Bethesda: NHLBI, 2007. Available from www.nhlbi.nih.gov/guidelines/asthma, last accessed 12 March 2013.

Scottish Intercollegiate Guidelines Network. *British Guideline on the Management of Asthma*, Guideline 101. Edinburgh: SIGN, 2008 (revised May 2011). Available from http://www.sign.ac.uk/pdf/qrg101.pdf, last accessed 12 March 2013.

Current therapies, particularly inhaled corticosteroids and long-acting bronchodilators, have excellent efficacy in controlling symptoms and preventing asthma exacerbations in nearly all people with asthma. In studies of asthma in the community, asthma symptoms are frequently poorly controlled, but this is most usually due to lack of availability of, or failure to take, recommended asthma controller therapies. However, not all patients achieve complete control of symptoms. For instance in a dose-escalation study using fluticasone dipropionate and salmeterol, only 72% of individuals achieved complete control of symptoms with high-dose inhaled therapy, although most of these had partially controlled asthma symptoms.

However, some individuals with asthma suffer from severe symptoms or may have progressive loss of lung function, together with frequent exacerbations despite optimal inhaled therapy. These individuals are considered to have refractory asthma.

Community studies of asthma severity suggest that approximately 5% of asthma sufferers have severe asthma and continue to suffer from uncontrolled asthma despite treatment. This group truly represent 'refractory' asthma and will fall into step 5 of the GINA treatment guidelines. International collaborative efforts are currently under way to study these individuals as they represent the major burden of asthma with respect to costs associated with emergency medical visits, hospitalizations and medications.

In considering whether a patient has 'refractory asthma' it is important not to escalate treatment without careful consideration of whether it is warranted. Three questions should be asked prior to diagnosing refractory asthma:

- Is the patient receiving their medication?
- Does the patient really have asthma?
- Does the patient have severe asthma?

## Is the patient receiving the medication?

Many obstacles exist to patients receiving and taking their medication. The degree to which a patient takes a medication as prescribed is termed 'adherence' and is an important goal of treatment for chronic diseases. It is estimated that fewer than 50% of individuals with an illness take medication exactly as prescribed.

Asthma medication may be difficult to obtain for reasons of cost or inconvenience. Asthma places a considerable burden on individuals and appears to be more common, and more severe, in lower income groups. The personal cost of asthma in terms of lost vocational opportunities, lost days at work and illness can be very significant and impair an individual's capacity to access and afford medical care. In some instances the financial burden of regular medication can exceed a patient's ability to pay for it. Patients can then decide not to take, or 'ration' asthma medication so that they receive less than was prescribed.

Non-adherence to medication can therefore be intentional due to economic reasons and other concerns surrounding medication use. Patients perform a 'cost–benefit' analysis as to whether to take prescribed medication, an analysis that includes their beliefs about the benefits of the treatment, its cost to them and the likely outcome of their asthma, and their fears about side effects (Figure 5.1). To address

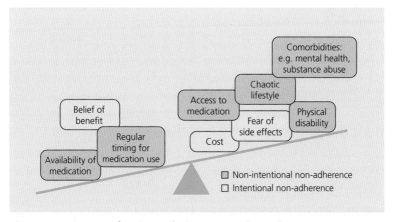

**Figure 5.1** Diagram of patient's decisions regarding adherence to medication: patients undertake a cost-benefit analysis of medication use.

intentional non-adherence, the health professional must take part in the patient's analysis and address issues that arise in order to aid adherence to a medication plan. This can be an excellent role for an asthma health educator.

People with asthma may also suffer from comorbidities that render it more difficult for them to acquire and take medication. For example, mental health issues and homelessness, where access to medication may be difficult and the lifestyle chaotic, will not be conducive to regular treatment use. This constitutes non-intentional non-adherence to medication and is dominantly driven by social and economic factors.

Once medication is prescribed and acquired, patients then need to use their device effectively. Many people, especially the young and very old, find the manipulation of inhaled devices difficult. A major part of consultation with a patient who is not successful in achieving good asthma control should be a review of inhaler use and technique, as this can be a significant barrier to effective treatment. Routinely, the substitution of a spacer device with an MDI can improve medication delivery and consequently asthma control. A further consideration is in those with low lung function and consequent poor inspiratory flows who may not reach required inspiratory flow to achieve drug deposition with dry powder devices.

So the first step in uncontrolled or poorly controlled asthma is the assessment of medication use and adherence. For the majority of individuals with uncontrolled asthma this will rectify the problem. In some instances measurement of blood corticosteroid levels can be performed, or dose counters used to formally assess adherence to medications where this is in doubt.

## Does the patient really have asthma?

Some diagnoses to consider are listed in Table 5.1. Important features on history are the onset of asthma, the presence of cough and sputum, a history of cigarette smoking and a history of infectious symptoms such as fever. Physical examination may point to a different pulmonary abnormality such as interstitial lung disease or pulmonary hypertension. In these instances chest imaging, such as an X-ray,

TABLE 5.1

**Other diagnoses to consider in refractory asthma**

- Vocal cord dysfunction
- Obesity
- Tracheal stenosis or compression
- Allergic bronchopulmonary aspergillosis
- Bronchiectasis
- Pulmonary hypertension
- Gastroesophageal reflux disease
- Chronic obstructive pulmonary disease
- Emphysema
- Interstitial lung disease

CT scan or echocardiography may be relevant. Allergic bronchopulmonary aspergillosis is a condition that complicates severe asthma due to airway colonization by fungi, leading to an exuberant immunologic response. Patients often present with fevers, cough and sputum as well as worsening asthma. Laboratory investigations including tests for blood specific immunoglobulin (Ig)E to *Aspergillus* spp. and total IgE are important in suggesting this diagnosis.

Any patient who does not respond to moderate doses of inhaled medication should undergo lung function testing to confirm a diagnosis of asthma. An obstructive deficit with reversibility should be documented. For children too young to perform spirometry reliably (usually under 7 years of age), a specialist opinion should be sought if the diagnosis is uncertain, as in children the consequences of unnecessary inhalation of corticosteroids (> 200 µg of HFA-beclometasone or equivalent per day) can be significant. Equally in adults, the use of frequent bursts of oral corticosteroids to control symptoms or the use of continuous oral corticosteroids should only be undertaken under specialist guidance.

## Does the patient have severe asthma?

A very few patients have severe asthma that continues to be unstable despite demonstrated reliable medication use. Such people should be referred to specialist care. These patients will often have abnormal lung function and also suffer from frequent exacerbations. They are usually managed using step 5 of the GINA guidelines for therapy. In this instance frequent continuous use of oral corticosteroids may be employed to achieve and maintain asthma control. As this will lead to side effects it is important that other available pharmaceutical options are employed. Long-term use of oral corticosteroids can be moderated by the use of steroid-sparing agents such as methotrexate or azathioprine, though these do not improve asthma control, only enable a reduction in corticosteroid dose. Frequent use of oral corticosteroids should trigger the monitoring of patients for common side effects of glucocorticoid use, such as diabetes and osteoporosis.

For patients with refractory asthma who have an allergic phenotype the drug omalizumab can be effective in reducing exacerbations and enabling a reduction in corticosteroid dose. Because of its expense, the use of omalizumab is usually confined to specialist centers. Other monoclonal antibody therapies have efficacy in refractory asthma and may also be employed, although their use is currently restricted to clinical trials (see Chapter 9).

**Non-invasive measurement of airway inflammation.** The presence of severe, refractory asthma is an indication for establishment of airway inflammatory phenotype. Cellular analysis of induced sputum can enable the diagnosis of eosinophilic airway inflammation which is much more likely to respond to corticosteroid treatments than a predominantly neutrophilic, or non-inflammatory sputum inflammatory pattern. Exhaled nitric oxide measurements may also be useful for the determination of the nature of airway inflammation, guiding further treatment options (see page 44). Treatment algorithms that use measures of airway inflammation suggest that there are some patients with high symptom burden but little evidence of inflammation: a dose reduction of anti-inflammatory therapies may be considered in this group (Figure 5.2).

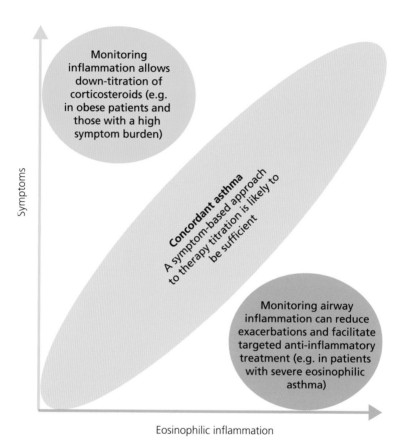

**Figure 5.2** In the majority of patients with asthma symptoms, exacerbations can be controlled with titration of inhaled therapy. Measurement of airway inflammation can facilitate treatment titration when asthma symptoms appear to be poorly controlled. Adapted from Haldar et al., 2008.

## Key points – refractory asthma

- Refractory asthma is characterized by uncontrolled symptoms and/or frequent exacerbations despite maximal inhaled medication including high-dose inhaled corticosteroids and long-acting beta-agonists.
- Refractory asthma is present in less than 5% of people with asthma.
- The first step in assessing refractory asthma is to assess adherence to current treatment.
- Before making a diagnosis of refractory asthma other conditions such as COPD and allergic bronchopulmonary aspergillosis should be excluded.
- Assessment of airway inflammation is a very useful step for guiding treatment in refractory asthma.

## Key references

Gamble J, Stevenson M, McClean E, Heaney LG. The prevalence of nonadherence in difficult asthma. *Am J Respir Crit Care Med* 2009;180:817–22.

Haldar P, Pavord ID, Shaw DE et al. Cluster analysis and clinical asthma phenotypes. *Am J Respir Crit Care Med* 2008;178:218–24.

Lotvall J, Akdis CA, Bacharier LB et al. Asthma endotypes: a new approach to classification of disease entities within the asthma syndrome. *J Allergy Clin Immunol* 2011; 127:355–60.

Asthma exacerbations remain one of the major causes of morbidity in asthma. They represent a significant burden of disease to patients and also to emergency healthcare providers. In children, asthma exacerbations remain one of the most common causes of school absence and hospital admission. In adults, exacerbations are responsible for loss of work time, emergency asthma attendances to primary care practitioners and hospital presentation and admission. A major indicator of risk for emergency asthma attendance is previous emergency attendance, indicating that preventive strategies should be applied for such individuals to prevent future severe and even life-threatening episodes. Fear of acute severe asthma is a major burden for many who live with severe asthma, and is a further reason for taking steps to prevent severe attacks.

## Patients at risk

Any patient with asthma can suffer from an acute asthma episode, often described as an asthma attack. Viral respiratory infections are the most common cause, accounting for at least 50% of hospital admissions for asthma in adults and over 80% in children. Such infections can be responsible for a rapid decline in lung function, which may not be entirely prevented by regular inhaled controller (preventer) therapy.

Other causes of acute asthma include acute allergen exposure, when an allergic person is exposed to an allergen not usually encountered in the environment. Examples of this include 'thunderstorm asthma' in people who usually have allergic rhinitis due to grass pollens, or individuals with allergy to molds. Inhalation of small allergen particles into the lower respiratory tract can cause a severe asthma episode and weather patterns can lead to epidemics of asthma in such circumstances. Similarly, severe food allergies (e.g. to peanuts or shellfish) may trigger asthma. While individuals with such a food allergy often present with signs of anaphylaxis, acute asthma is a major component of a severe food reaction for some and it requires recognition and treatment in its own right.

Some medications, such as β-blockers – even in eye drops – may also be responsible for an acute exacerbation of asthma. Individuals with acetylsalicylic acid (ASA; aspirin)-sensitive asthma may have severe asthma after taking ASA or other non-steroidal anti-inflammatory drug (NSAID) that has cyclooxygenase (COX)-1 activity such as indometacin, ibuprofen, naproxen, piroxicam, and nabumetone. The mechanism probably relates to inhibition of formation of protective prostaglandins such as prostaglandin $E_2$ (PGE$_2$). COX-2 inhibitors such as celecoxib are much less likely to cause reactions. NSAID reactions are most often described in individuals with non-allergic asthma who have nasal polyposis. Individuals with this type of asthma should avoid ASA and preferably all NSAIDs, although if absolutely necessary (e.g. a patient with severe rheumatoid arthritis and asthma), a supervised trial of a COX-2 inhibitor might be considered. It is important to be aware of other preventable causes of exacerbations such as occupational and sometimes unusual allergen exposures.

Regular use of controller asthma medication substantially reduces, but does not completely eliminate, the risk of an acute asthma attack. Asthma exacerbations may occur in individuals with asthma who do not receive adequate controller treatment. All individuals who present with an acute exacerbation should be asked what controller treatment they are taking, and consideration should be given to introducing or adjusting regular maintenance medication in order to prevent such exacerbations in the future.

## Recognizing a severe attack

It is important for patients and clinicians alike to recognize the signs of a severe asthma attack and know when to seek further help.

**Patients** can recognize a severe asthma attack by the frequency and severity of symptoms (Figure 6.1). Asthma symptoms that recur and require bronchodilator treatment more frequently than once every 4 hours are an indication of an attack that requires medical treatment.

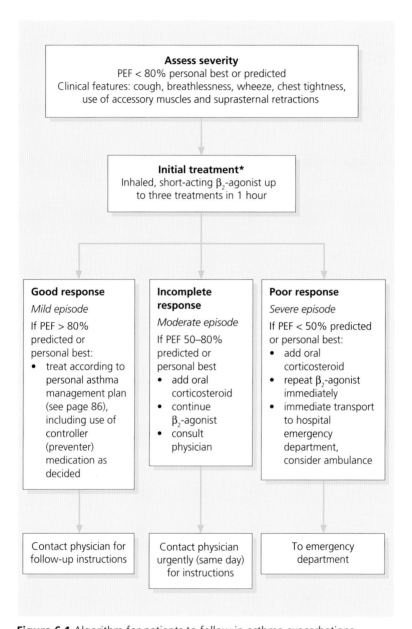

**Assess severity**
PEF < 80% personal best or predicted
Clinical features: cough, breathlessness, wheeze, chest tightness,
use of accessory muscles and suprasternal retractions

**Initial treatment***
Inhaled, short-acting β$_2$-agonist up
to three treatments in 1 hour

**Good response**

*Mild episode*

If PEF > 80%
predicted or
personal best:
• treat according to
  personal asthma
  management plan
  (see page 86),
  including use of
  controller
  (preventer)
  medication as
  decided

**Incomplete response**

*Moderate episode*

If PEF 50–80%
predicted or
personal best
• add oral
  corticosteroid
• continue
  β$_2$-agonist
• consult
  physician

**Poor response**

*Severe episode*

If PEF < 50% predicted
or personal best:
• add oral
  corticosteroid
• repeat β$_2$-agonist
  immediately
• immediate transport
  to hospital
  emergency
  department,
  consider ambulance

Contact physician for
follow-up instructions

Contact physician
urgently (same day)
for instructions

To emergency
department

**Figure 6.1** Algorithm for patients to follow in asthma exacerbations.
*Patients at high risk of asthma-related death should contact a physician
promptly after initial treatment as additional therapy may be required.
PEF, peak expiratory flow.

Most often, patients with a severe exacerbation of asthma describe their asthma as being 'out of control'. This is a clear sign that urgent help is needed. Patients may also monitor their peak expiratory flow (PEF). A measurement of 50% of predicted or less that does not respond promptly to bronchodilator treatment is an indication for seeking emergency help.

**Clinicians** should assess the severity of an acute attack of asthma according to Table 6.1. It is important to remember that asthma severity is classified according to the worst parameter.

Features to observe are respiratory rate, state of consciousness and whether the patient is able to speak in full sentences, phrases or in words. All patients presenting to a doctor with an acute exacerbation of asthma must be assessed objectively for airflow obstruction by PEF measurement, or by blood gas measurement if PEF measurement is not possible.

## Management by the patient

Patients with asthma should have a personal written asthma action plan that provides information to aid recognition of an acute attack and lists treatment options (see Chapter 6). Action plans should include a crisis plan, and explain when it is appropriate for a patient to call an ambulance. Plans must be written individually for each patient, but generally patients should seek urgent medical help if they have used reliever medication three or more times without response, if they feel out of control or if their PEF remains below 50% of predicted.

For less severe attacks that do not require hospital presentation, the first step is to increase regular bronchodilator therapy (however, frequent symptoms and frequent requirement for bronchodilator suggest that further treatment is needed). Less severe asthma attacks are diagnosed by frequent requirement for bronchodilator (up to once every 4 hours), night waking with asthma and breathlessness. As a rule, the PEF will be 50–80% of predicted, with the range depending on the person's asthma history. Oral corticosteroids, that is

prednisolone, 1 mg/kg or 50 mg daily for adults, may be initiated by the patient in consultation with a primary care practitioner. For those with more severe asthma, prompt access to a supply of oral corticosteroids is important to prevent severe exacerbations, and such patients may keep a store of these medications at home. Once started, oral corticosteroid therapy should be continued for at least 5 days.

## Hospital referral

Hospital referral is indicated for all patients who have persisting severe asthma or symptoms despite oral corticosteroid therapy and for those in whom asthma is severe (see Figure 6.1). Patients with a history of severe or brittle (unpredictable and severe) asthma, intensive care admission, difficulties in accessing care or psychosocial problems may require hospital referral at an earlier stage. Admission to hospital enables the administration of parenteral asthma therapy and observation of a patient with severe airflow obstruction to ensure there is a response to asthma treatment, thereby ensuring patient safety. The hospital also provides an environment for ventilatory support if this is required.

Most deaths of people with asthma occur out of hospital, usually in those with severe chronic asthma but also in some considered to have mild asthma. Treatment with bronchodilator medication in the absence of controller (preventer) treatments or overuse of bronchodilator medication is a particular risk factor for fatal asthma. Further risk factors are a previous life-threatening asthma attack, admission to hospital for asthma in the previous year and social or physical isolation from medical care, including psychosocial disability, especially psychiatric illness, substance abuse, poor treatment adherence and difficulty accessing treatment. Individuals with these features should be observed carefully and may require early referral to hospital.

Protective factors for asthma death are regular use of inhaled corticosteroids and possession of a personal written asthma management plan.

All patients who have been admitted to hospital with asthma should see a respiratory specialist. Those with life-threatening or brittle asthma should remain under the care of a specialist.

TABLE 6.1

**Classification of severity of asthma exacerbations (the presence of several signs, but not necessarily all, can be used to indicate the severity of an asthma exacerbation)**

| Characteristic | Mild | Moderate |
|---|---|---|
| Breathless | When walking | When talking<br>Infants: softer, shorter cry, difficulty feeding<br>Can lie down |
| Speech: talks in… | Sentences | Phrases |
| Alertness | May be agitated | Usually agitated |
| Respiratory rate[†] | Increased | Increased |
| Accessory muscles and suprasternal retractions | Usually not | Usually |
| Wheeze | Moderate, often only end-expiratory | Loud |
| Pulse[‡] | < 100 bpm | 100–200 bpm, depending on age |
| PEF[§] after bronchodilator (% predicted or personal best) | > 80% | Approximately 60–80% |
| $PaO_2$ (on air) | Normal; test not usually necessary | > 60 mmHg |
| and/or $PaCO_2$ | < 45 mmHg | < 45 mmHg |
| $SpO_2$ (on air) | > 95% | 91–95% |

*Any of the listed features indicate a severe episode.
[†]Normal rates in children: < 2 months, 60 breaths/minute; 2–12 months, < 50 breaths/minute; 1–5 years, < 40 breaths/minute; 6–8 years, < 30 breaths/minute.
[‡]Normal rates in children: 2–12 months, < 160 bpm; 1 year, < 120 bpm; 2–8 years, < 110 bpm.
[§]Children ≤ 7 years old are unlikely to be able to perform PEF readings reliably.

| Severe* | Respiratory arrest imminent |
|---|---|
| At rest<br>Infants: stops feeding | |
| Prefers sitting | Hunched forwards |
| Words | |
| Usually agitated | Drowsy or confused |
| Often > 30 breaths/minute | |
| Usually | Paradoxical thoracoabdominal movement |
| Usually loud but may become silent | Absent |
| Usually > 120 bpm in adults 120–200 bpm in children, depending on age | Bradycardia |
| < 60% (< 200 liters/minute in adults), or bronchodilator response lasts < 2 hours | Patients with very severe asthma are unlikely to able to perform PEF readings reliably |
| < 60 mmHg; possible cyanosis | |
| > 45 mmHg; possible respiratory failure | |
| < 90% | |

bpm, beats per minute; $PaCO_2$, partial pressure of carbon dioxide in arterial blood; $PaO_2$, partial pressure of oxygen in arterial blood; PEF, peak expiratory flow; $SpO_2$, oxygen saturation estimated by pulse oximetry.

## Treatment of acute severe asthma in hospital

Treatment of an acute exacerbation is based on the initial assessment of severity. Classification of severity depends on objective signs of airflow obstruction, including ability to talk in sentences, pulse rate, conscious state and, most importantly, PEF readings. Oxygen saturation measurements are useful, but it is important to remember that an oxygen saturation result may be elevated by oxygen administration with nebulized medication and does not reflect the adequacy of ventilation as determined by blood $CO_2$ measurements.

**In the emergency department.** The principles of acute asthma management in the emergency department are outlined in Figure 6.2. All patients should receive inhaled bronchodilator, and those with moderate or severe exacerbations should receive oral or parenteral corticosteroid therapy. For patients with life-threatening attacks, intensive care services should be sought. Patients not responding to treatment and stable within 2 hours should be considered for admission to hospital.

**In hospital.** Acute asthma management in hospital is summarized in Figure 6.3. Once a patient is admitted to hospital, monitoring and treatment should continue with:

- frequent (at least every 2 hours) observation of PEF, oxygen saturation, blood pressure and pulse
- oxygen administration to maintain oxygen saturation above 92%
- administration of $\beta_2$-agonists at least every 4 hours, and continuously if required
- administration of corticosteroid therapy orally or intravenously
- observation for deterioration in clinical state.

For asthma exacerbations, 8–12 puffs of a $\beta_2$-agonist with a spacer device is approximately equivalent to 5 mg of salbutamol delivered by a nebulizer. This method of short-acting $\beta_2$-agonist delivery may be preferred for reasons of infection control or community use. Familiarity with the delivery of salbutamol by metered-dose inhaler (MDI) and spacer will also assist people with asthma and their carers to deliver care for asthma exacerbations following discharge from hospital.

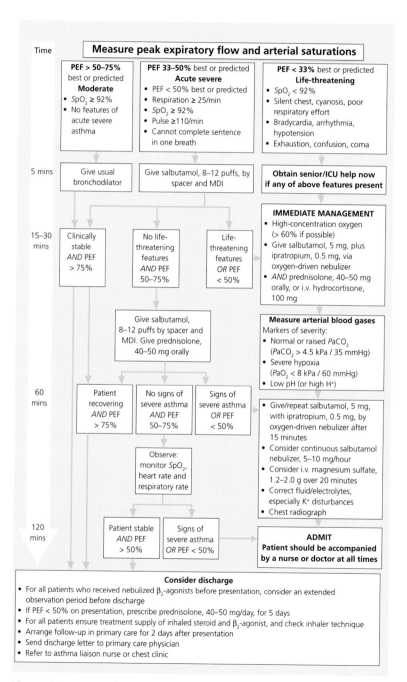

**Figure 6.2** Acute asthma management in the emergency department.

### Day 1 Admission to ward

**Monitor:**
- HR, BP, $SpO_2$, PEF at least every 2 hours unless determined otherwise by medical staff

**Medications all patients receive:**
- Oxygen to maintain $SpO_2$ > 92%
- Salbutamol, 8–12 puffs, by spacer and MDI every 2–4 hours or salbutamol, 5 mg, and ipratropium, 0.5 mg, by nebulizer every 4 hours
- Hydrocortisone, 100 mg i.v., every 6 hours
- If salbutamol infusion commenced, continue at 5–20 µg/minute

### At all stages

**Test arterial blood gases if:**
- Elevated $PaCO_2$ at previous estimate (repeat test within 2 hours unless PEF has improved to > 50% predicted)
- Decline in $SpO_2$ to < 92%
- Decline in PEF to < 50% predicted
- Deterioration in conscious state
- Confusion
- Patient distressed

### Admission to intensive care if:
- Worsening hypoxia, hypercapnia or acidosis
- Increasing exhaustion
- Deterioration in conscious state, confusion

- Monitor HR, BP, $SpO_2$, PEF at least every 4 hours unless determined otherwise by medical staff
- Check $SpO_2$ on air daily if safe; cease supplemental $O_2$ when $SpO_2$ > 92% on air
- Daily review by medical staff, review medications
- Review maintenance asthma medications
- Initiate asthma education
- Daily fingerprick blood glucose level
- Check U&E on day 2; repeat at least daily if abnormal

### Consider discharge when:
- Medication review steps 1–4 accomplished
- Symptoms substantially improved
- PEF improved to > 75% of previous best or predicted
- Patient is stable and has been maintained on oral and inhaled medication for at least 12 hours

### At discharge ensure:
- Patient has written asthma management plan
- Patient has begun the education process
- Follow-up appointment arranged within 2 weeks
- Discharge summary sent to primary care physician

### Medication review as determined by patient condition:
1. Wean from nebulized salbutamol to MDI and spacer
2. Substitute i.v. hydrocortisone with oral prednisolone, 50 mg per day
3. Commence high-dose inhaled corticosteroid therapy, e.g. beclometasone or budesonide, 200–400 µg twice daily, fluticasone propionate, 250–500 µg twice daily, fluticasone furoate, 250 mg twice daily, or ciclesonide, 320 µg daily.
4. Replace regular $\beta_2$-agonist with 'as required' $\beta_2$-agonist (via a MDI)

**Figure 6.3** Algorithm for management in the hospital ward of adults with acute asthma. BP, blood pressure; HR, heart rate; MDI, metered dose inhaler; $PaCO_2$, partial pressure of oxygen in arterial blood; PEF, peak expiratory flow; $SpO_2$, oxygen saturation estimated by pulse oximetry; U&E, urea and electrolytes.

Ongoing review in hospital ensures recovery and introduces patients to their ongoing preventative medication and the management plan likely to be required following a hospital admission for asthma. The time in hospital presents an ideal opportunity for formal asthma education; interventions that provide in-hospital asthma education have shown benefits in terms of reduced re-admission rates.

## Follow-up

All patients should leave hospital with medication, a written plan of what to do if their asthma worsens and a follow-up medical appointment for ongoing management. Oral corticosteroid therapy should be continued for at least 5 days following hospital discharge. It is important that asthma control is assessed following a hospital admission and that ongoing maintenance medication is adjusted accordingly.

### Key points – acute asthma attacks

- Asthma exacerbations are one of the major causes of morbidity in asthma, resulting in loss of work time in adults or school absence in children, and emergency hospital presentation and admission.
- Causes of acute asthma include viral respiratory infections, acute allergen exposure, food allergies and some medications such as acetylsalicylic acid (aspirin) and non-steroidal anti-inflammatory drugs.
- Acute exacerbations of asthma usually respond well to inhaled $\beta_2$-agonists and a course of oral corticosteroid.
- After hospital admission, patients should receive appropriate medication, a written plan of what to do if their asthma worsens and a follow-up medical appointment for ongoing management and measurement of lung function.

## Key references

Goeman DP, Aroni RA, Sawyer SM et al. Back for more: a qualitative study of emergency department reattendance for asthma. *Med J Aust* 2004;180:113–17.

Global Initiative for Asthma. *Global Strategy for Asthma Management and Prevention; Updated 2012.* Available from www.ginasthma.org, last accessed 12 March 2013.

Scottish Intercollegiate Guidelines Network. *British Guideline on the Management of Asthma*, Guideline 101. Edinburgh: SIGN, 2008 (revised May 2011). Available from www.sign.ac.uk/pdf/qrg101.pdf, last accessed 12 March 2013.

Preventing asthma attacks is the most effective means of controlling asthma. Effective prevention involves identifying and avoiding risk factors and asthma triggers, together with effective patient education and adherence to a medication regimen.

## Patient partnerships

Included in the goals of good asthma management is the need to meet patients' goals and expectations as well as those of the health practitioners. Good asthma management means that a partnership should be established between the patient and health professional, with shared treatment goals noted in a jointly written and agreed self-management plan. This eases the pressure on healthcare personnel resources by helping patients to take responsibility for their health and improves asthma outcomes.

## Risk factor avoidance

Identifying the risk factors that trigger asthma attacks and removing the appropriate allergens and irritants from the patient's environment can reduce the frequency of symptoms and hospitalizations for asthma, and the need for medication. Appropriate avoidance behaviors are shown in Table 7.1. However, allergens should only be avoided when there is evidence that the patient is indeed allergic to that specific allergen. Patients with a true allergy will have both a history of symptoms on exposure to an allergen and immunologic evidence of sensitivity, for example a positive skin-prick test or blood-specific immunoglobulin (Ig)E test. If these are not present then allergen avoidance is not recommended.

**House dust mites** are the most common source of domestic allergens. They breed rapidly in damp humid climates. Avoidance measures should be particularly directed at the patient's bedroom, but ideally the entire home should be treated. Bed linen and blankets should be

TABLE 7.1

**Allergen and irritant avoidance**

**Allergen avoidance**

*House dust mite*

- Wash bed linen and blankets once a week in hot water (> 55°C)
- Protect mattresses and pillows with air-tight covers
- Remove carpets, particularly in bedrooms
- Avoid fabric-covered furniture
- Wash curtains and soft toys
- If possible, use a vacuum cleaner with filters

*Animal allergens*

- Remove animals from house
- If removal of family pets is not possible or desirable, keep animals out of bedrooms and wash the animal regularly

*Cockroach allergen*

- Clean infected houses regularly
- Use pesticides (but ensure asthmatic patient is not present if pesticide sprays are used, and air house thoroughly before patient returns)

*Fungal spores and pollens*

- Close doors and windows and remain indoors when mold and pollen counts are highest
- Air conditioning can be helpful providing the unit is kept clean

**General measures**

*Tobacco smoke*

- Stop smoking
- Avoid smoking in rooms used by children with asthma
- Avoid public areas where people smoke

CONTINUED

TABLE 7.1 (CONTINUED)

*Indoor air pollutants*

- Vent all furnaces and stoves to exterior
- Keep rooms well ventilated
- Avoid household sprays and polishes

*Colds and other viral respiratory infections*

- Patients with asthma should have annual influenza vaccination
- When cold symptoms appear, treat with inhaled short-acting $\beta_2$-agonist, introduce oral corticosteroids early, or increase inhaled corticosteroid dose if asthma status deteriorates
- Continue anti-inflammatory treatment for several weeks to ensure adequate control

*Physical activity*

- Should not be avoided, but appropriate medication is necessary:
  - pretreat with short- or long-acting $\beta_2$-agonist or cromoglicate before exercising
  - training and warm-up exercises can reduce symptoms

washed weekly in hot water, and mattresses and pillows protected by air-tight covers. Carpets and furnishing fabrics should be avoided wherever possible, and the bedroom should be well ventilated. Acaricides are of little use. Unfortunately, even with these measures it is difficult to reduce the concentrations of domestic mite allergens below the threshold that induces symptoms in allergic individuals.

**Animal allergens.** A pet in the home to which the patient with asthma is allergic is a major risk factor for current asthma symptoms. Ideally, such pets – usually cats – should be removed from the home, but this may not be acceptable. If animals cannot be removed, they should be kept away from bedrooms; weekly washing of the pet appears to reduce the allergen load but may be poorly tolerated by the animal. Other animals that are particularly allergenic are rodents (mice, rats and guinea pigs) and horses.

**Cockroach allergen** is a major cause of asthma in some areas, particularly in inner city environments. It can be reduced by regular cleaning of the home and by the use of pesticides. If pesticide sprays are used, however, the patient should not be present while spraying is in progress, and the home should be aired thoroughly before the patient returns.

**Molds and pollens.** The number of fungal spores can be reduced by removing or cleaning mold-infested objects. A low humidity (less than 50%) is important, and so a dehumidifier or air conditioning may be useful; such devices should be cleaned regularly. Exposure to outdoor allergens, such as pollens, can be minimized by keeping doors and windows closed, and by remaining indoors as much as possible during high-risk periods.

**Smoking.** Passive smoking increases the risk of allergic sensitization in children and worsens the frequency and severity of symptoms in asthmatic children. Parents of such children should be advised not to smoke and to prohibit smoking in rooms used by their children.

**Indoor pollutants.** Common indoor pollutants include nitrogen dioxide, carbon monoxide and particles. Adequate ventilation and maintenance of heating systems are the most effective measures for reducing exposure to such pollutants.

**Occupational exposure.** Early identification of occupational sensitizers and removal of the patient from further exposure are important elements in the management of occupational asthma.

**Food allergy** is a rare cause of asthma exacerbations and may occur at any age. Individuals with severe food allergies should avoid the food in question and be assessed by an allergy specialist. Clear evidence of IgE immunoreactivity to the food or a positive double-blind food challenge should be obtained to justify and clarify the role of ongoing food avoidance. Patients with both asthma and severe food allergies causing anaphylaxis are at particular risk of severe attacks and death.

They should be well educated in the avoidance of the specific food and should have access to autoinjectable epinephrine (adrenaline), such as the EpiPen.

**Acetylsalicylic acid (ASA; aspirin) intolerance** is an important cause of worsening asthma in adults. Patients who are affected should be advised to avoid all non-steroidal anti-inflammatory drugs (NSAIDs) except those selective against cyclooxygenase-2 (COX-2).

## Treatment of rhinitis

Symptoms of rhinitis include a runny, itchy or blocked nose and there may also be sneezing and symptoms of eye irritation and tiredness. Rhinitis is more common than asthma, and international surveys reveal that its prevalence appears to be increasing. The prevalence of asthma is increased in those with both allergic and non-allergic rhinitis by two- to fivefold, and 80% of individuals with asthma suffer from symptoms of rhinitis. It is increasingly evident that effective treatment of rhinitis can assist in the management of asthma. Regular use of topical nasal corticosteroids is the recommended treatment for all but mild intermittent rhinitis. Topical nasal corticosteroid therapy for rhinitis in those with concurrent asthma in addition to regular controller asthma therapy can nearly halve the risk of asthma exacerbations requiring emergency treatment. Allergen immunotherapy can also be an effective treatment for severe or refractory allergic rhinitis, and an associated improvement in asthma outcomes has been shown.

## Immunotherapy

Specific immunotherapy, aimed at treating the underlying allergy, has been shown to be effective in patients with asthma caused by house dust mite, grass or other pollens, and animal dander. Such treatment may be useful in patients for whom allergen avoidance is not possible or whose symptoms are poorly controlled by conventional medication, or where a single allergen is especially problematic. Allergen immunotherapy is usually delivered by subcutaneous or sublingual

99

routes by a specialist medical practitioner. Considerable effort is now being spent on improving the tolerogenicity of allergens and reducing their anaphylactogenic effects. This type of treatment probably works by inducing a subset of regulatory T lymphocytes (Treg) that secrete inhibitory cytokines such as interleukin (IL)-10 and transforming growth factor (TGF)β. However, there is increasing evidence to support the use of sublingual immunotherapy. As immunotherapy is relatively contraindicated in those with unstable asthma and those with abnormal lung function, it is practically limited to those with milder disease, especially those who suffer from allergic rhinitis. There is some evidence that immunotherapy can prevent the progression of allergic rhinitis to asthma.

Immunotherapy should only be undertaken by healthcare professionals with specific training in the diagnosis of allergy and the management of anaphylaxis.

## Asthma management plans

Education is essential to enable patients to make the decisions needed to control their asthma. This involves the preparation of a detailed management plan (Table 7.2), which is agreed between the patient and the physician, and is tailored to the needs and circumstances of the individual patient. Plans based on symptoms or on measurement of peak expiratory flow (PEF) have been shown to be equally effective. Plans should be written down so patients can refer to them (Figures 7.1 and 7.2).

A zone system, which classifies the level of asthma control according to symptoms and PEF (if available), is a useful feature of management plans. This approach helps patients to understand the chronic and variable nature of asthma, monitor their condition, identify signs of deteriorating control and take appropriate action.

**Traffic-light plan.** In the management plan shown in Figure 7.1, the three zones correspond to the colors of a traffic light.

*The green zone* indicates 'all clear'. Asthma is controlled, with few symptoms (less than two a week) and no interference with everyday life; PEF is 80–100% of personal best and PEF variability is less than

TABLE 7.2

**Elements of an asthma management plan**

- The daily dose of long-term preventive medication needed to control asthma and prevent symptoms
- Specific triggers to avoid
- What to do if asthma worsens:
  - name and dose of bronchodilator to be taken immediately for quick relief of symptoms
  - how to recognize deteriorating control (e.g. increasing cough, chest tightness or breathing difficulties, nocturnal symptoms, increasing use of quick-acting reliever medicine)
  - how to treat worsening asthma, and what to do if a cold develops
  - how and when to seek medical attention

20%. Moving to a lower treatment step can be considered if the patient remains in this zone for at least 3 months.

*The yellow zone* indicates that caution is necessary. Mild symptoms are present and PEF is 60–80% of personal best with 20–30% variability. This may indicate an acute attack requiring a temporary increase in medication, or an overall deterioration that requires additional treatment.

*The red zone* indicates an emergency. Asthma symptoms are present at rest and may interfere with activity; PEF is below 60% of personal best. Immediate intervention is necessary.

**Credit-card-sized plan.** Another management plan, the credit-card-sized document shown in Figure 7.2, has been evaluated in clinical trials, and has been successfully introduced in several countries, including the UK, New Zealand and Australia.

## Promoting adherence

Patients' asthma will not be controlled effectively if they do not adhere to their medication and management plan, yet adherence studies reveal

## Asthma management plan

Think about the colors of a traffic light to learn about your asthma medication.

**Red** means **Stop**
Get help from a doctor

**Yellow** means **Caution**
Use quick-relief medicine

**Green** means **Go**
Use preventive medicine

Name: _____
Doctor: _____ Date: _____
Telephone no. for doctor or clinic: _____
Telephone no. for taxi or friend: _____

### 1. Green – Go

- Breathing is good
- No cough or wheeze
- Can work and play

Peak flow number
............ to ............

**Use preventive medicine**

| Medicine | How much to take | When to take it |
|---|---|---|
| | | |
| | | |
| | | |
| 20 minutes before sport use this medicine | | |
| | | |

### 2. Yellow – Caution

- Wheeze
- Cough
- Tight chest
- Wake up at night

Peak flow number
............ to ............

**Take quick-relief medicine to keep an asthma attack from getting bad**

| Medicine | How much to take | When to take it |
|---|---|---|
| | | |
| | | |
| | | |
| | | |

### 3. Red – Stop – Danger

- Medicine is not helping
- Breathing is hard and fast
- Nose opens wide
- Can't walk
- Ribs show
- Can't talk well

Peak flow number
............ to ............

**Get help from your doctor now**
Take these medicines until you talk with the doctor

| Medicine | How much to take | When to take it |
|---|---|---|
| | | |
| | | |
| | | |
| | | |

**Figure 7.1** Asthma management plans can be based on a zone system, with action needed to control asthma at different levels of severity.

that fewer than 50% of patients take their medication as prescribed. Causes of non-adherence may be intentional or non-intentional. Intentional non-adherence is the result of a balancing consideration that patients make about their medications (see Figure 5.1). Other reasons why patients choose not to take a medication may be unrelated to the medication (Table 7.3).

Regular consultations are necessary to give patients an opportunity to talk about their concerns, needs and expectations in relation to

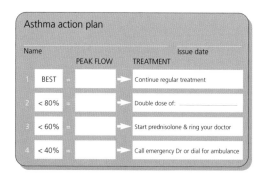

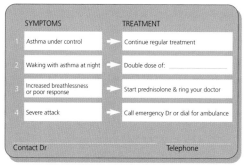

**Figure 7.2** A credit-card-sized asthma self-management plan. This plan has been evaluated in clinical trials and introduced in several countries.

their asthma and its treatment. Action can then be taken to address any problems identified, and to resolve any fears or concerns that patients may have. Strategies for encouraging adherence are listed in Table 7.4. Recent evidence supports the use of digital technology such as mobile phone reminder systems, mobile applications (apps) to assist in asthma management and MP3 messages to improve asthma awareness and knowledge.

Together, the patient and the healthcare professional can identify joint goals of treatment, such as 'staying out of hospital', 'attending school camp' or 'playing football', that are relevant to the patient and likely to promote adherence. At each visit, the physician should check:

• whether the stated goals have been achieved
• adherence to, and concerns about, medication and the management plan
• the patient's use of the controller (preventer) and reliever inhalers, PEF meter or other devices
• need for emergency attendances
• avoidance of triggers.

TABLE 7.3

**Factors leading to non-adherence with asthma therapy**

**Medication-related factors**

- Misunderstanding the need for both long-term and short-acting drugs
- Complicated treatment regimens
- Difficulty in giving medicine to young children
- Difficulty using inhalers
- Adverse effects
- Fear of adverse effects or addiction
- Cost
- Dislike of medication
- Distance to pharmacies

**Non-medication factors**

- Disbelief or denial of cause of symptoms or attacks
- Misunderstanding of management plan
- Lack of guidance for self-management
- Dissatisfaction with healthcare professionals
- Fears or concerns not expressed or discussed
- Inappropriate expectations
- Poor supervision, training or follow-up
- Cultural issues (traditions, beliefs about asthma and its treatment)
- Family issues (e.g. smoking, pets)
- Forgetfulness or complacency when non-symptomatic
- Chaotic lifestyle, (e.g. substance abuse, homelessness)

Once control has been achieved, regular follow-up every 1–6 months is necessary to assess whether the management plan is meeting its objectives. This includes an assessment of asthma control, including:

- nocturnal symptoms
- the effect of symptoms on normal activity

TABLE 7.4

**Strategies for improving adherence to asthma treatment**

- Enquire about adherence to medication (patients are generally honest in admitting non-adherence)
- Educate patients and their families about the inflammatory basis of asthma and the need for ongoing treatments
- Enquire about and address concerns regarding medications and their use
- Identify and, if possible, address barriers to medication use (e.g. cost, knowledge of how to use the devices)
- Ask about family and cultural beliefs
- Encourage the patient in self-management
- Keep medication regimens simple – twice a day maximum
- Explain likely side effects and how to prevent them
- Be positive about the outcomes of treatments
- Plan for regular medical review at least twice a year
- Discuss measures that will help patients get in the habit of regular inhaler use, such as:
  - a regular time of use, e.g. before or after meals or after brushing your teeth
  - keeping your inhaler in plain sight where it will prompt use (e.g. next to the coffee pot)
  - asking a family member or friend to help you remember to take your medication
  - putting sticky-note reminders in obvious places (e.g. on the fridge)
  - using technology to provide reminders (e.g. text alerts, watch alarms)

- use of reliever rescue medication
- need for urgent medical attention
- spirometry or peak flow reading.

Trained asthma educators may also be used to help patients acquire knowledge about their asthma and to address concerns that prevent use of controller medications. There is evidence that asthma education can improve outcomes of patients admitted to hospital with asthma.

## When to refer

In general, most patients with mild or moderate asthma can be adequately managed in the primary care setting. Referral to a specialist is advisable for patients with moderate or severe persistent asthma, those reaching step 5 of the GINA management guideline and those with complicating conditions or circumstances (Table 7.5). Children needing more than 200 µg inhaled HFA-beclometasone or the daily equivalent of inhaled corticosteroid, and adults needing more than 1000 µg per day with poor symptom control, should also be referred to a specialist.

TABLE 7.5

**Situations requiring specialist referral for asthma**

- Life-threatening attacks
- Moderate or severe persistent asthma
- Patient is unable to cope with self-management
- Atypical signs or symptoms, or difficulties with differential diagnosis
- Complicating conditions such as sinusitis, nasal polyposis, aspergillosis or severe rhinitis
- Further diagnostic tests required (e.g. provocation testing or complete lung function tests)
- Patient does not respond optimally to treatment
- Additional guidance needed (e.g. trigger avoidance or treatment complications)

## Key points – preventing asthma attacks

- Preventing asthma attacks is the most effective means of controlling asthma.
- Identifying risk factors that trigger asthma attacks and removing allergens and irritants from the patient's environment can reduce the frequency of symptoms and hospitalizations for asthma, and decrease the need for medication.
- Immunotherapy is helpful in some patients when one of the following applies:
  - specific allergens can be shown to be causative
  - allergen avoidance is not possible
  - symptoms are not controlled by conventional medication.
- A written self-management plan empowers patients to manage their asthma optimally.
- Failure to respond to treatment may result from non-adherence to the prescribed treatment. Attention must be paid to the patient's ability to take their inhaled therapy correctly. Identifying problems surrounding care and creating a patient partnership with agreed treatment goals can facilitate adherence.

## Key references

Abramson MJ, Puy RM, Weiner JM. *Cochrane Database Syst Rev* 2010;(8):CD001186.

Brozek JL, Bousquet J, Baena-Cagnani CE et al. Allergic rhinitis and its impact on asthma (ARIA) guidelines: 2010 revision. *J Allergy Clin Immunol* 2010:126:466–76.

Gibson PG, Powell H, Wilson A et al. Self-management education and regular practitioner review for adults with asthma. *Cochrane Database Syst Rev* 2003;(1): CD001117.

Global Initiative for Asthma. www.ginasthma.org

Mosnaim GS, Cohen MS, Rhoads CH et al. Use of MP3 players to increase asthma knowledge in inner-city African–American adolescents. *Int J Behav Med* 2008;15:341–6.

## 8  Exercise-induced asthma

Up to 80% of people with asthma will develop exercise-induced symptoms, so that exercise for some people is a real trigger for their asthma. Indeed, in some people asthma is only evident on exercising; this is particularly the case for children, in whom the benefits of exercise are especially important. Consequently, managing exercise-induced asthma and enabling individuals to exercise despite asthma is an important part of asthma management.

In addition, the issue of asthma in elite sporting activities has risen to prominence. In some Olympic teams as many as 20% of athletes declare that they have asthma, raising concerns about the appropriate use of anti-asthma medications in this group. Optimizing asthma diagnosis and treatment in elite athletes is critical to optimizing performance and deserves particular attention.

### Diagnosis

Exercise-induced asthma is defined as a transient increase in airway resistance that follows vigorous exercise. Many people complain of shortness of breath while exercising, and this symptom is often magnified in people with asthma. A history of developing wheeze, shortness of breath and sometimes cough both during and after exercise should prompt a clinician to consider a diagnosis of exercise-induced asthma. Exercise-induced asthma is particularly common in children and approximately 80% of children with asthma will have evidence of exercise-induced bronchoconstriction. For some individuals with brittle asthma, the response to exercise can be severe and may be a strong disincentive to exercise.

Exercise-induced asthma appears to be more common in those with allergies to inhaled substances and often occurs on exercise in very cold weather. A feature of exercise-induced asthma is a refractory period, whereby induction of exercise-induced asthma appears to be protective for further episodes for a period of several hours. Thus, individuals who experience a bout of exercise-induced asthma can undertake subsequent exercise with relative protection from further episodes. Some people with asthma use this strategy to manage exercise-induced symptoms by undertaking a warm-up to exercise of short, high-intensity exercise bursts. The refractory period can be inhibited by anti-inflammatory medications such as indometacin.

For most, exercise-induced asthma can be diagnosed on symptoms or wheeze or excess dyspnea during or following exercise, which may be confirmed with peak flow testing. However, in some cases it is important to make a diagnosis of exercise-induced asthma so, in the lung function laboratory or for research purposes, exercise-induced asthma can be brought on by a short period (6–8 minutes) of high-intensity exercise of at least 70% of maximum capacity. Lung function is measured following this exercise; a decline in the forced expiratory volume in 1 second ($FEV_1$) of more than 10% from baseline denotes a diagnosis of exercise-induced asthma (Figure 8.1).

## Mechanisms

During inhalation air is humidified and warmed to body temperature. At rest, this process usually occurs in the upper airways, particularly

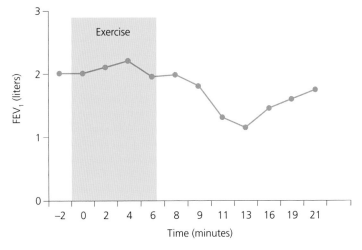

**Figure 8.1** Exercise challenge testing: during brief high-intensity exercise lung function transiently improves, but lung function is likely to fall in the minutes following exercise in people with exercise-induced asthma.

109

in the nose. During exercise, ventilation is increased, sometimes to levels exceeding 100 L/min, so that the individual has to breathe through the mouth to overcome upper airway resistance. Mouth breathing and increased ventilation lead to recruitment of the lower airways to warm and humidify inspired air, resulting in progressive evaporation of airway surface fluid and consequent hyperosmolarity of this fluid. It is thought that hyperosmolarity of the airway surface fluid provokes mast cell degranulation, which can then stimulate airway narrowing through smooth muscle contraction. In support of these theories, exercise-induced asthma has been shown to correlate with increased blood, lavage and urinary mast cell mediators. In addition, breathing humidified warmed air during exercise has been shown to be protective for the development of exercise-induced bronchoconstriction. Swimming is often recommended as an exercise to people with asthma, as inspiration will occur from the humidified air near the water surface, decreasing the dehydrating stimulus to the lower airways.

By contrast, many individuals with asthma find cold air a potent trigger of symptoms. This is because the water content of air is temperature dependent, cold air holding less water than warmer air. Thus, exercise in the cold, such as skiing, requires greater water transfer for complete saturation of inspired air than does exercise in warmer climates, and cold dry air is therefore a more potent stimulus for developing exercise-induced asthma.

Exercise-induced symptoms appear to be more common in atopic individuals; this observation may imply that inhaled allergens play a role. In particular, loss of the protective functions of the upper airways during inspiration may permit increased penetration to the lower respiratory tract of allergens and other particles likely to stimulate asthma. Although this has not been proven to be a cause in laboratory-induced exercise-induced asthma, increased lower airway exposure to allergens and extremes of environmental changes such as heat and cold may be particularly relevant in elite athletes who spend a large amount of time training with high ventilation, thereby increasing their cumulative exposure to such potential triggers.

## Airway challenge for the diagnosis of exercise-induced asthma

The problem with laboratory exercise tests is that they may not replicate the environmental conditions under which exercise is performed. For example, neither the temperature nor the humidity of ambient air is likely to be the same as that encountered during outdoor exercise. In addition, it is often difficult to achieve adequately high workloads for very fit individuals, such as athletes, using laboratory exercise equipment. Hence, field testing can be undertaken to make the diagnosis, which requires recording of peak expiratory flow (PEF) or lung function following exercise in the field. However, this too is subject to varying conditions of humidity, temperature and conduct of the test, rendering standardization difficult. As a consequence of these difficulties, surrogate challenges for exercise-induced asthma have been developed so that a diagnosis can be consistently achieved.

**Airway challenge testing** can be categorized into direct and indirect airway responses (Figure 8.2). Indirect challenges cause bronchoconstriction by stimulating airway mast cells to release mediator and thereby cause secondary airway smooth muscle constriction. Direct challenges act pharmacologically on the airway smooth muscle to cause airway narrowing.

*Indirect challenges.* Exercise challenge testing is an indirect challenge relying on airway responses to exercise, such as airway drying and cooling, to cause smooth muscle contraction. Because of the difficulties of replicating field exercise in the laboratory to achieve consistency of diagnosis, a number of surrogate challenges for exercise have been developed. Chief among these is the eucapnic voluntary hyperventilation challenge, in which the individual is asked to breathe a mixture of dry air with 5% carbon dioxide at 85% of their maximal ventilation (approximately 30 times $FEV_1$) for 6 minutes, and their $FEV_1$ is monitored after challenge. This surrogate challenge has been shown to correlate very well with actual exercise challenge and is suitable for use by athletes. A fall in $FEV_1$ of 10% following the eucapnic voluntary hyperventilation challenge has been adopted by the

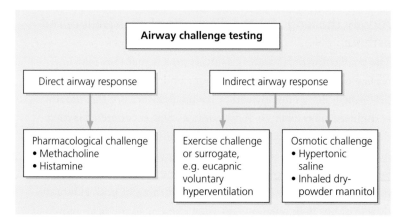

**Figure 8.2** Airway challenge tests for direct and indirect airway responses.

International Olympic Committee as the preferred criterion for confirmation of an asthma diagnosis in elite athletes.

Indirect airway challenges such as mannitol and hypertonic saline have been shown to correlate very well with eucapnic voluntary hyperventilation challenges. These agents mimic the dehydration of the airways that is probably responsible for exercise-induced asthma.

*Direct challenges.* Most individuals with airway hyperresponsiveness to methacholine will yield a positive result to exercise challenge. However, some – particularly elite – athletes will have a positive surrogate exercise challenge result despite negative direct airway challenge test results. It is therefore important not to exclude exercise-induced asthma on the basis of a negative direct airway challenge test result.

## Exercise-induced asthma in athletes

The high prevalence of exercise-induced asthma in elite athletes has been an issue of concern. Escalating use of bronchodilator treatments by elite athletes has prompted rulings from the International Olympic Committee so that diagnosis of asthma in elite competition must be confirmed by lung function abnormality or challenge testing. Some elite cold-weather athletes, such as cross-country skiers, are very likely to develop exercise-induced asthma (so called 'skier's asthma'). In summer athletes, a high occurrence of asthma has been reported in elite swimmers. In both these instances, training for prolonged periods at high ventilatory workloads and consequent high exposure to very cold or chlorinated air, respectively, is thought to contribute to an airway injury that may lead to exercise-induced asthma. The finding that older athletes and those from sports that are predominantly aerobic are more likely to have exercise-induced asthma supports this theory.

The symptoms of elite athletes with asthma are thought to differ from those of non-athletes in that they may complain of poor performance or fatigue rather than dyspnea. Investigation of symptoms of elite athletes revealed that traditional asthma symptoms have a sensitivity of only 60% in predicting exercise-induced bronchoconstriction in laboratory challenge. Thus, poor performance in an athlete ought to prompt consideration of exercise-induced asthma. The diagnosis of exercise-induced asthma in elite athletes must be verified by airway challenges. Eucapnic voluntary hyperventilation and mannitol are both suitable challenges for this purpose.

## Treatment

Treatment for exercise-induced asthma in those with pre-existing asthma is determined by evaluating lung function and symptoms. Individuals with lung function abnormalities and symptoms of asthma both with and without exercise should have the usual controller (preventer) medication prescribed. Inhaled corticosteroids have been shown to be very effective in reducing airway hyperresponsiveness both generally and following exercise. However, many people with asthma do have asthma symptoms despite regular use of inhaled corticosteroids and may require additional short-acting $\beta_2$-agonists (SABAs) before exercise to prevent exercise-induced asthma.

Some individuals with normal interval lung function complain of symptoms only on exercise. Although regular preventive treatment may be appropriate for such people if exercise is very frequent, it may be reasonable to use SABAs to prevent exercise-induced bronchoconstriction in those who experience symptoms only episodically, such as less than twice a week. Additional or alternative treatments may be required in some, and include mast cell stabilizers such as cromoglicate or nedocromil, or leukotriene modifiers such as montelukast.

Non-drug strategies for the treatment of exercise-induced asthma rely on the refractory period that follows induction of airway narrowing with exercise. It is frequently recommended that athletes with exercise-induced asthma warm up slowly. They may institute strategies such as repeated high-intensity runs during a warm-up to prevent exercise-induced asthma occurring in the main competition.

**Key points – exercise-induced asthma**

- Exercise-induced asthma is defined as a transient increase in airway resistance that follows vigorous exercise.
- It appears to be more common in those with atopy and to be seen more often on exercise in very cold weather.
- Induction of exercise-induced asthma appears to be protective for further episodes for a period of several hours.
- Exercise testing or other direct or indirect challenges are used in diagnosis.
- In elite athletes, direct airway challenges may not reveal exercise-induced asthma, so indirect surrogate challenges must be used to confirm diagnosis.
- First-line treatment of exercise-induced asthma is inhaled corticosteroids to reduce airway hyperresponsiveness, with additional short-acting $\beta_2$-agonists before exercise if necessary.

**Key references**

Fitch KD, Sue-Chu M, Anderson SD et al. Asthma and the elite athlete: summary of the International Olympic Committee's Consensus Conference, Lausanne, Switzerland, January 22–24, 2008. *J Allergy Clin Immunol* 2008;122:254–60.

Holzer K, Anderson SD, Douglass J. Exercise in elite summer athletes: Challenges for diagnosis. *J Allergy Clin Immunol* 2002;110:374–80.

The future looks most promising for patients with asthma. But until new treatments are developed, it is essential that we make better use of the drugs currently available.

## Preventive immunologic treatments

The incidence of allergy and asthma in developing countries has increased with the acquisition of westernized lifestyles. It has been suggested that this observed increase may be due to the decreasing incidence of childhood infections and other environmental influences such as alteration in diet and intestinal bacterial flora. Immune stimulation by infections in early life may be necessary for the differentiation of T regulatory lymphocytes which can modulate immune responses. Observations that a rural lifestyle appears to offer some protection from allergic diseases may support this theory. The role of dietary manipulation early in life to prevent allergic disease is still the subject of intense interest, with large-scale cohort studies under way.

Studies are also under way to attempt to manipulate the responses to allergens early in life to facilitate the development of regulatory immune responses. These include trials of mycobacterial vaccines and probiotics.

Allergen immunotherapy is a productive area for developments in this arena. Some evidence exists that allergen immunotherapy can prevent the development of asthma in those with allergic rhinitis. Increasing attention is being devoted to the development of safer forms of injected allergen immunotherapy and more convenient modes of sublingual administration of allergen immunotherapy extracts.

In addition, intensive research is focused on developing a safer form of inhaled corticosteroid that interferes with the inflammatory pathways underpinning the pathogenesis of asthma and yet does not produce the usual side effects.

## Assessing airway inflammation

The development of methods of measuring the underlying airway inflammation in asthma heralds changes in the choice of asthma treatments. The most commonly used non-invasive method of establishing the nature of airway inflammation is induced sputum analysis for cells, which is cumbersome to incorporate into daily clinical practice. The refinement of this and other methods of quantifying airway inflammation – such as measurement of exhaled gases, particularly exhaled nitric oxide – may be more convenient and allow more precise direction of treatments. Better definition of asthma inflammatory phenotype enables delivery of treatments that target a specific underlying type of inflammation and has particular relevance in the delivery of therapies addressing a specific type of asthma.

## Severe asthma

As severe asthma constitutes a major part of burden of asthma to the health system, further developments in asthma treatments are particularly focusing on those with difficult-to-treat asthma. Two recent studies support the effectiveness of specific monoclonal antibodies in severe asthma and provide evidence that in this group of patients, treatments should be directed to airway inflammatory subtypes (see above).

These monoclonal antibody treatments (see below) are particularly effective in individuals with eosinophilic airway inflammation that fails to respond to corticosteroid treatment. Currently there are no proven effective therapies for individuals with asthma with predominantly neutrophilic airway inflammation. While macrolide antibiotics or statin therapies may hold promise for these patients, the results of trials are awaited. Newer therapies such as phosphodiesterase inhibitors are also being developed in this area.

**Mepolizumab** is a humanized monoclonal antibody that binds to interleukin (IL)-5. IL-5 is a potent activator, chemoattractant and growth factor for eosinophils. This drug has been shown to be effective in reducing exacerbations in those patients with severe, refractory eosinophilic asthma. As with omalizumab, mepolizumab is likely to be indicated for those asthma patients who have failed to respond to maximal doses of inhaled medication. Mepolizumab is given by a monthly intravenous dose. While large clinical trials are currently progressing, this medication offers promise for those patients with severe refractory disease. Mepolizumab is also the first medication directed to those with a specific subtype of asthmatic airway inflammation, namely eosinophilic asthma; early trials in asthma patients undifferentiated by airway inflammation failed to reveal efficacy.

**Lebrikizumab** is a humanized monoclonal antibody binding to, and neutralizing, IL-13. This cytokine is released by Th2 lymphocytes and is likely to play a role in stimulating the airway wall remodeling associated with asthma. Administration of this antibody improved lung function in individuals with inadequately controlled asthma. Those who demonstrated improvement had higher blood levels of periostin, a factor induced from bronchial epithelial cells by IL-13; this may indicate an inflammatory subtype of asthma particularly likely to benefit from this antibody therapy.

**Bronchial thermoplasty** uses locally applied heat, delivered by bronchoscope, to diminish the amount of airway smooth muscle and therefore reduce bronchial hyperresponsiveness. Consequently it may be particularly useful in individuals with severe airway hyperresponsiveness. Current evidence appears positive in reducing airway hyperresponsiveness and asthma symptoms, but evidence of long-term outcomes is awaited.

## Genetic targeting

As treatments become more geared towards total prevention and cure of asthma, it is likely that they will focus not on broad populations, but on individuals who are at specific genetic risk. Many asthma genes have been identified, and although certain genes that increase the risk either of having asthma or of having more severe disease have been identified, it is likely that many more will be found that are more important and are, therefore, of direct relevance in selecting patients for appropriate treatments.

The results of genetic studies are also likely to have an impact on drug treatment, as polymorphisms involving cellular receptors or enzyme pathways against which drugs are directed may influence their effectiveness (pharmacogenetics).

## Key references

Anderson GP. Endotyping asthma: New insights into key pathogenic mechanisms in a complex, heterogeneous disease. *Lancet* 2008;372:1107–19.

Castro M, Musani AI, Mayse ML, Shargill NS. Bronchial thermoplasty: a novel technique in the treatment of severe asthma. *Ther Adv Respir Dis* 2010;4:101–16.

Corren J, Lemanske RF, Hanania NA et al. Lebrikizumab treatment in adults with asthma. *N Engl J Med* 2011;365:1088–98.

Haldar P, Brightling CE, Hargadon B et al. Mepolizumab and exacerbations of refractory eosinophilic asthma. *N Engl J Med* 2009;360:973–84.

Pavord ID, Korn S, Howarth P et al. Mepolizumab for severe eosinophilic asthma (DREAM): a multicentre, double-blind, placebo-controlled trial. *Lancet* 2012;380:651–9.

Woodruff PG, Modrek B, Choy DF et al. T-helper type 2-driven inflammation defines major subphenotypes of asthma. *Am J Respir Crit Care Med* 2009; 180:388–95.

# Useful resources

## UK

Asthma UK
Tel: +44 (0)20 7786 4900
Helpline: 0800 121 62 44
info@asthma.org.uk
www.asthma.org.uk

British Lung Foundation
Tel: +44 (0)20 7688 5555
Helpline: 03000 030 555
www.blf.org.uk

British Thoracic Society
Tel: +44 (0)20 7831 8778
bts@brit-thoracic.org.uk
www.brit-thoracic.org.uk

The James Lind Alliance
Working Partnership in Asthma
www.lindalliance.org/Asthma_
Working_Partnership.asp
patkinson@lindalliance.org
Tel: +44 (0)1865 517 635

Scottish Intercollegiate
Guidelines Network (SIGN)
www.sign.ac.uk/guidelines/fulltext/
101/index.html

## USA

Allergy & Asthma Network
Mothers of Asthmatics
Tel: 1 800 878 4403
www.aanma.org

American Academy of Allergy,
Asthma & Immunology
Tel: +1 414 272 6071
info@aaaai.org
www.aaaai.org

American Association for
Respiratory Care
Tel: +1 972 243 2272
info@aarc.org
www.aarc.org

American Lung Association
Tel: +1 202 785 3355
Helpline: 1 800 586 4872
www.lung.org

Asthma and Allergy Foundation
of America
Toll-free: 1 800 727 8462
info@aafa.org
www.aafa.org

US Environmental Protection
Agency
www.epa.gov/asthma

**International**

**Allergic Rhinitis and its Impact on Asthma**
www.whiar.org

**The Asthma Foundation (New Zealand)**
Tel: +64 (0)4 499 4592
info@asthmafoundation.org.nz
www.asthmanz.co.nz

**European Academy of Allergy and Clinical Immunology**
Tel: +41 44 205 55 33
info@eaaci.net
www.eaaci.net

**European Federation of Allergy and Airway Diseases Patients' Association**
Tel: +32 (0)2 227 2712
info@efanet.org
www.efanet.org

**Global Initiative for Asthma**
www.ginasthma.org

**International Union Against Tuberculosis and Lung Disease**
Tel: +33 (0)1 44 32 03 60
www.theunion.org

**The Lung Association (Canada)**
Tel: +1 613 569 6411
Toll-free: 1 888 566 5864
info@lung.ca
www.lung.ca

**National Asthma Council Australia**
Tel: +61 (0)3 9929 4333
Toll-free: 1 800 032 495
nac@nationalasthma.org.au
www.nationalasthma.org.au

**PatientPictures.com**
www.patientpicutres.com/resp
Includes clinical drawings on asthma – allergen avoidance, diagnosis, symptoms and treatments

**Thoracic Society of Australia & New Zealand**
Tel: +61 (0)2 9222 6200
info@thoracic.org.au
www.thoracic.org.au

# FastTest – Now Test Yourself ...

## 1  Pathophysiology

i. What are the two principal manifestations of disordered lung function in asthma?

ii. What four mechanisms are responsible for reduced airflow in asthma?

iii. Name four predisposing risk factors for asthma.

## 2  Epidemiology and natural history

Are the following statements true or false?

i. High doses of short-acting $\beta_2$ agonists (SABAs) have been associated with increased mortality in asthma.

ii. Lung growth may be reduced in children with severe persistent symptoms of asthma.

iii. Regular use of corticosteroids in early life alters the natural history of asthma.

## 3  Diagnosis and classification

i. Name four clinical signs of asthma.

ii What $FEV_1$ and PEF results, taken before and after inhalation of a SABA are indicative of asthma?

iii. Name five risk factors associated with an increased risk of death from asthma.

## 4 Management

i. What are the main aims of asthma management?

ii. Name two anti-inflammatory and two reliever therapies.

iii. How long should asthma treatment remain on a particular management step before escalation or reduction?

## 5 Refractory asthma

i. What three questions should be asked prior to diagnosing refractory asthma?

ii. What differential diagnoses should be considered in patients with refractory asthma?

iii. When is a cellular analysis of induced sputum particularly useful?

## 6 Acute asthma attacks

Are the following statements true or false?
i. Viral respiratory tract infections are the most common cause of hospital admissions in acute asthma.
ii. Protective factors for asthma death include regular use of SABAs.
iii. Oral corticosteroid therapy should be continued for 5 days following discharge from hospital.

## 7  Preventing asthma attacks

i. Name four measures to avoid exposure to house dust mite.

ii. Apart from house dust mite, what other common allergens have the potential to trigger an asthma attack?

iii. Name five ways in which you can help patients adhere to their asthma treatment.

## 8  Exercise-induced asthma

Are the following statements true or false?

i. Exercise-induced asthma appears to be protective against further episodes for a period of several hours.

ii. Exercise-induced asthma can be diagnosed only by measuring lung function during high-intensity exercise.

iii. All individuals who experience exercise-induced asthma should be prescribed controller (prevention) medication and a reliever inhaler.

# ... The Answers

**1 Pathophysiology**
i.   The two principal manifestations of disordered lung function in asthma are bronchial (airway) hyperresponsiveness and airflow limitation (or airflow obstruction). (p10)
ii.  The four mechanisms responsible for reduced airflow in asthma are acute bronchoconstriction, swelling of the airway wall, chronic mucous plug formation and airway wall remodeling. (p10, Table 1.1 and pp11–12)
iii. Predisposing risk factors for asthma include genetic predisposition, atopy, airway hyperresponsiveness, sex, race/ethnicity and family size. (p15, Table 1.3)

**2 Epidemiology and natural history**
i.   True: SABAs have been associated with increased mortality in asthma when used without anti-inflammatory treatments. (p27)
ii.  True: Lung growth may be reduced in children with severe persistent symptoms of asthma. (p33)
iii. False: There is no evidence that regular use of corticosteroids in early life alters the natural history of asthma. (p33)

**3 Diagnosis and classification**
i.   Clinical signs of asthma include breathlessness, speaking in words, increased respiratory rate, wheezing (although a silent chest may indicate life-threatening obstruction), hyperinflation (hunched shoulders, use of accessory muscles or preferring not to lie down), cough, tachycardia, associated conditions (e.g. eczema, rhinitis), cyanosis, drowsiness and a reduced peak flow reading less than 80% of predicted normal. (pp38–41, Table 3.2)
ii.  A 12% or 200 mL (whichever is greater) improvement of $FEV_1$, or more than 15% or at least 60 L/min improvement in PEF, 15 minutes after SABA inhalation, indicates asthma. (pp40–1, Table 3.3)
iii. Factors associated with an increased risk of death from asthma include: a previous history of acute life-threatening attacks, psychosocial problems, hospitalization for asthma within the previous year, a history of invasive ventilation for asthma, recent reduction or cessation of systemic corticosteroid therapy, non-adherence to preventive treatments and difficulty accessing treatment. (p50)

**4 Management**
i.   The main aims of asthma management are control of symptoms, prevention of exacerbations, maintenance of pulmonary function as close to normal levels as possible, maintenance of normal levels of activity, prevention of the development of irreversible airflow limitation and prevention of asthma mortality. (p52, Table 4.1)
ii.  Anti-inflammatory medications include inhaled corticosteroids (e.g. beclometasone dipropionate, budesonide, fluticasone propionate), systemic corticosteroids (e.g. prednisolone), leukotriene modifiers (e.g. zafirlukast, montelukast), sodium cromoglycate and nedocromil sodium, and omalizumab. (pp52–8)
     Reliever medications include SABAs (e.g. salbutamol, terbutaline), LABAs with a rapid onset of action (e.g formoterol), systemic corticosteroids, anticholinergic drugs (e.g. ipratropium bromide) and short-acting theophylline. (pp58–60)
iii. Depending on the severity of symptoms, treatment should be continued at the same level for 1–3 months before considering escalation or reduction. (p69)

**5 Refractory asthma**
i.   The three questions to ask before diagnosing refractory asthma are: Is the patient receiving their medication (adherence)? Does the patient really have asthma (differential diagnoses)? Does the patient have severe asthma? (pp76–80)
ii.  Differential diagnoses for refractory asthma include vocal cord dysfunction, obesity, tracheal stenosis or compression, allergic bronchopulmonary aspergillosis, bronchiectasis,

pulmonary hypertension, gastroesophageal reflux disease, chronic obstructive pulmonary disease, emphysema and interstitial lung disease. (p79, Table 5.1)

iii. Cellular analysis of induced sputum is particularly useful in patients with severe refractory asthma who remain unstable despite reliable medication use. Eosinophilic inflammation is more likely to respond (than predominantly neutrophilic inflammation) to corticosteroid treatment. (p80)

**6 Acute asthma attacks**

i. True: Viral respiratory tract infections are the most common cause of hospital admissions in acute asthma (accounting for at least 50% of cases in adults and over 80% in children). (p83)

ii. False: Protective factors for asthma death include regular use of inhaled corticosteroids and a personal written asthma management plan. (p87)

iii. True: Oral corticosteroid therapy should be continued for at least 5 days following discharge from hospital. (p93)

**7 Preventing asthma attacks**

i. Measures to avoid exposure to house dust mite include: washing bed linen and blankets once a week in hot water (> 55°C), protecting mattresses and pillows with airtight covers, removing carpets, especially in the bedroom, avoiding fabric-covered furniture, washing curtains and soft toys, and if possible using a vacuum cleaner with filters. (pp95–7, Table 7.1)

ii. Common allergens with the potential to trigger an asthma attack include animal allergens, cockroach allergen, fungal spores and pollens. (pp96–8, Table 7.1)

iii. Ways in which you can help patients adhere to their asthma treatment include: ask about adherence; educate about the inflammatory basis of asthma and the need for ongoing treatment; discuss concerns regarding drugs and their use; identify barriers to medication use; encourage self-management; keep medication regimens simple; explain side effects and how to prevent them; be positive about outcomes; review regularly (at least twice a year); discuss habit-forming measures. (p105, Table 7.4)

**8 Exercise-induced asthma**

i. True: A feature of exercise-induced asthma is a refractory period, which enables individuals to undertake subsequent exercise with relative protection from further episodes. (pp108–9)

ii. False: In most cases, exercise-induced asthma can be diagnosed from symptoms of wheeze or excess dyspnea during or following exercise and can be confirmed with peak flow testing. (p109)

iii. False: It may be reasonable to use only a SABA to prevent exercise-induced asthma in individuals who experience symptoms episodically (e.g. less than twice a week). (p113)

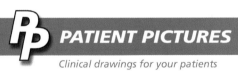

# Index